To read

Before becoming

Night nursing

assistant

MARTIN STERLING

Table of contents

Chapter 7: Risk and Safety Management in the Night Shift   121

« *Working at night means watching over lives when the world is asleep, bringing comfort and care in the shadows, where every gesture counts double, because it's done in silence and solitude. It's a vocation that requires inner strength and unwavering empathy, because to be a night orderly is to be the light that guides patients through the darkest hours.* »

Chapter 1
Introduction
Night Service
in Care

- **The importance of night work in hospitals**
  - ◦ **Organizing night-time care**

The organization of night-time care in a healthcare facility is a complex process that relies on meticulous planning, close coordination between members of the care team, and anticipation of patients' specific needs during the night. Unlike daytime hours, when hospital activities are more intense and a multitude of professionals are present, nighttime imposes a reduced workforce and a different distribution of tasks, making every action particularly crucial.

One of the fundamental aspects of the organization of night-time care is the handover, a key moment when the day team transmits to the night team all the necessary information on the patient's state of health, the care in progress, and any emergencies to be anticipated. This transmission must be exhaustive and precise, as it determines the quality of care provided throughout the night. By receiving this information, orderlies prepare themselves to manage care autonomously, while being ready to call on the assistance of the nurse or doctor on duty if necessary.

At night, the main objective of care is to ensure continuity and safety for patients, while respecting their need for rest. Care is therefore planned to be as non-disruptive as possible. Care assistants ensure that rounds are carried out regularly, with particular attention to the most vulnerable patients, such as those in intensive care, the elderly or patients at the end of life. During these rounds, they monitor vital signs, check on patients' comfort, and ensure that their basic needs are met.

Administering medication is also an important part of the night. It must be carried out with the utmost precision, as fatigue can impair caregivers' vigilance. Protocols are therefore rigorous, and each caregiver is trained to follow medical prescriptions scrupulously, while being able to detect and report any signs of distress or adverse reactions.

At the same time, the organization of night-time care includes the management of emergencies. Even if emergencies are statistically less frequent at night, their occurrence is often more critical, due to the reduced availability of human and technical resources. Nursing assistants must therefore be particularly responsive and capable of mobilizing the necessary resources quickly, while maintaining effective communication with the medical team.

The relational dimension is not overlooked in the organization of night-time care. At night, patients may experience heightened feelings of loneliness, anxiety or discomfort, amplified by silence and darkness. Nurses play a crucial role in providing psychological support, offering a reassuring presence, responding to emotional needs and helping patients through difficult times.

Finally, the organization of night-time care must also take into account the needs of the caregivers themselves. Working at night imposes a different pace of life, which is often physically and mentally demanding. Team managers must therefore ensure that caregivers have the necessary breaks to recuperate and maintain their vigilance throughout their shift. Strategies to support and prevent fatigue-related risks are also put in place, to safeguard the health and well-being of staff.

○   **The crucial role of the night orderly**

The role of the night orderly is of paramount importance in the operation of healthcare establishments. While the day is marked by intense activity and the presence of numerous healthcare professionals, the night imposes a different framework where silence, darkness and reduced staffing levels create an atmosphere where every gesture counts double. In this context, the night orderly becomes a central figure, ensuring continuity of care, the safety of patients, and the emotional support they need in moments of vulnerability.

Although often less visible than their daytime colleagues, night nurses have essential responsibilities that go far beyond technical tasks. They are the guarantors of continuity of care. When the day teams hand over, it's up to the night carer to ensure that each patient continues to receive the care he or she needs, whether it's pain management, monitoring vital signs, or comfort care. This requires constant vigilance and the ability to work independently, as direct medical resources are often more limited at night.

With this autonomy comes the need for initiative and judgment. The night orderly is often called upon to rapidly assess situations, recognize early warning signs of deterioration in a patient's state of health, and decide what action needs to be taken urgently. For example, if a patient presents symptoms of respiratory distress or acute pain, the caregiver must not only intervene immediately to relieve the patient, but also alert the nurses or doctor on duty. This front-line role, combined with the ability to alert quickly when needed, makes the caregiver a key element of the night care safety system.

Over and above the technical and supervisory aspects, night nurses also play a fundamental role in the human accompaniment of patients. The night is a time when loneliness, fear and anxiety can become more prevalent, especially among the most fragile patients or those in critical situations, such as palliative care. The caregiver then becomes a reassuring presence, an attentive ear capable of soothing and comforting. He or she must know how to listen, reassure, and sometimes simply be there, so that the patient feels safe and less alone in the face of his or her nocturnal worries.

In addition, the night orderly contributes to maintaining a calm, restful care environment, which is essential for patient recovery. He or she must ensure that the course of care is as undisturbed as possible, while being attentive to each patient's individual needs. This may include simple but essential gestures, such as readjusting a pillow, bringing a glass of water, or simply making sure the patient is comfortable for the night.

Night work also requires the caregiver to develop specific skills, such as fatigue and stress management, as staggered working hours can have an impact on physical and mental health. They must therefore be able to maintain constant vigilance and efficiency throughout the night, while recognizing their own limitations and asking for help if necessary. This resilience is essential if we are to deliver quality care despite the challenges inherent in night-time work.

Finally, the night orderly has a key role to play in passing on crucial information to the day shift. They must be able to effectively communicate observations made during the night, the care provided, and any notable events that occurred during their shift. This fluid communication ensures that patients continue to receive the best possible care, with no break in their care.

- ◦ **Specific features of night shifts compared with day shifts**

Compared to the day shift, the night shift has specific features that make it unique and demanding, both in terms of organization and care. These particularities stem from a combination of factors linked to the circadian rhythms of caregivers and patients, downsizing, the general atmosphere of the hospital, and the types of care and interventions required during the night. Understanding these specifics is essential if we are to fully appreciate the challenges and responsibilities of working at night in a hospital environment.

One of the main differences between day and night shifts lies in the rhythm and nature of activities. During the day, hospital wards are animated by a multitude of interventions: consultations, examinations, surgical procedures, doctors' visits, and paramedical activities. Daytime services are characterized by an intensity of activity that mobilizes a large number of healthcare professionals, enabling rapid, diversified patient care. By contrast, the night shift is characterized by a relative calm, marked by a reduction in planned interventions and a general decrease in noise and agitation. This apparent tranquility, however, does not mean a reduction in responsibilities. On the contrary, it requires caregivers to demonstrate heightened vigilance and the ability to intervene quickly when needed, often with fewer resources available.

Another major feature of night shifts is the reduction in the number of staff. Night shifts are generally smaller, with fewer nurses, doctors on call, and orderlies. This downsizing calls for a rigorous organization of work, with each team member needing to be versatile and capable of managing a variety of situations independently. Night carers, particularly orderlies, are therefore often required to take the initiative and demonstrate a high degree of autonomy in managing care. They must be prepared to take on a greater share of responsibility, whether for monitoring patients, responding to their urgent needs, or identifying signs of deteriorating health that require immediate intervention.

The night shift is also distinguished by the atmosphere in the hospital. At night, silence and darkness transform the hospital environment. This special setting influences not only patients, but also caregivers. For patients, nighttime can exacerbate feelings of anxiety, loneliness and vulnerability. Fears often manifest themselves more intensely, particularly in the elderly, patients at the end of life, or those suffering from cognitive disorders. Night carers therefore need to develop a particular sensitivity to these psychological aspects, and be prepared to offer increased emotional support, as a complement to physical care. Their role is to create a reassuring environment, soothe anxieties, and provide a caring presence that mitigates the potentially anxiety-provoking effects of the night.

In terms of care, the specific features of night-time care call for an approach tailored to the needs of patients during this period. Priority is often given to comfort care and monitoring, in order to respect patients' sleep while ensuring their safety. Night rounds are essential to check on patients without waking them unnecessarily. Care must be planned to disrupt rest as little as possible, while remaining sufficiently frequent to prevent complications. For example, the prevention of pressure sores in bedridden patients requires special attention, as does pain management, which may occur more intensely at night and require immediate intervention so that the patient can continue to rest.

Finally, nocturnal emergencies, although less frequent, are often more critical. At night, in the absence of daytime hustle and bustle, every emergency situation must be managed with maximum efficiency and speed, despite the limited availability of resources. Night nurses must be particularly responsive, able to call in the right people quickly and manage the situation until they arrive. This dimension reinforces the importance of collaboration and communication within the night team, where everyone must be able to rely on each other to ensure optimal patient care.

- **Motivations for choosing night work**
  - ◦ **Challenge and vocation**

Challenge and vocation are at the heart of a caregiver's professional life, especially for those who work night shifts. This profession, often overlooked by the general public, represents much more than a simple occupation: it embodies a genuine commitment, a call to devote oneself to others at the most crucial moments of their lives. This vocation is inseparable from the many challenges that caregivers face every day, night after night, in a demanding and often difficult environment.

The challenge begins as soon as the caregiver takes on his or her role, a role that demands great physical and mental resilience. Working the night shift imposes a different rhythm on life, disrupting the body's natural cycle and requiring constant adaptation. Fatigue, isolation and the silence of the night can take a heavy toll on morale, but it is precisely in these conditions that the caregiver must remain vigilant, alert and ready to intervene at a moment's notice. This daily challenge is compounded by the need to manage often complex situations with greater autonomy, as shifts are smaller and resources more limited during the night. Every decision taken, every action undertaken, must be measured and effective, because the margins for error are slim, and the consequences can be significant.

Over and above the physical and organizational aspects, the challenge for the caregiver also lies in coping with the most difficult human realities. At night, patients are often more vulnerable, and their fears and suffering more present. The caregiver must therefore not only provide technical care, but also offer a comforting presence, an emotional support that is essential to soothe the anguish and loneliness that patients may feel. This "night watchman" role is a demanding one, requiring constant empathy, the ability to listen, and a willingness to offer comfort at what can be a very delicate time.

This is where vocation comes in. Without this inner strength, without this deep desire to serve and care for others, the challenge of night work could quickly become insurmountable. Vocation is what gives meaning to every gesture, to every night spent looking after others. It is the driving force that pushes the caregiver to get up every night, to face up to fatigue, stress and difficulties in order to be where he or she is most needed. This vocation is often fuelled by deep-seated values: altruism, the desire to contribute to the well-being of others, and the conviction that every act of care, however humble, can make a difference to patients' lives.

The night orderly thus embodies a total commitment, where challenge and vocation combine to give meaning to a demanding but profoundly human profession. It is in this duality that the night orderly finds his strength: the challenge pushes him to surpass himself, to develop his skills and resilience, while the vocation gives him the energy and motivation to persevere, night after night. This unique combination makes the night orderly not only a skilled professional, but also a dedicated person, ready to stand by patients in the darkest moments of their lives.

◦ **The advantages and disadvantages of night shifts**

Night duty, with its particularities and demands, presents both advantages and disadvantages that shape the experience of those who choose this path. For care assistants, these contrasting aspects combine with both the daily challenge and the vocation that drives them, creating a professional landscape that is as rewarding as it is complex.

One of the major advantages of a night shift is that the work rhythm is often perceived as calmer than during the day. At night, the hospital or healthcare establishment enters a sort of standby mode, where scheduled interventions are less frequent, and the general atmosphere is more peaceful. For some caregivers, this setting offers a valuable opportunity to focus more on the well-being of patients, to have more personalized interactions, and to deliver care with greater attention. This relative calm makes it possible to develop a close relationship with patients, responding to their needs with more time and compassion, away from the hustle and bustle of the day.

Another advantage is the possibility of better remuneration. Night shifts are often paid at a premium, providing financial compensation for working odd hours. This can be particularly attractive for those looking to maximize their income while balancing their professional and personal lives. What's more, night duty can offer a degree of flexibility in the organization of the day, allowing caregivers to attend to personal or family matters during the hours when most people are working.

However, with these advantages come a number of disadvantages that can weigh heavily over time. The main drawback of night shift work is undoubtedly the impact on physical and mental health. Working against one's natural biological rhythm can lead to sleep disorders, chronic fatigue, and even increased risk of cardiovascular and metabolic diseases. The human body is not naturally designed to stay awake at night, and this inversion of cycles can have significant long-term repercussions. Fatigue accumulated night after night can also affect alertness, concentration and the ability to provide optimal care, posing a risk to both caregiver and patient.

Social isolation is another notable disadvantage. Working at night often means being out of touch with those around you, which can limit social interaction and affect family relationships. Time shared with family and friends is less frequent, and it can be difficult to maintain a fulfilling social life when you have to sleep during the day. This isolation can lead to a feeling of loneliness and remoteness, making night work sometimes emotionally difficult to bear.

On a professional level, the night shift can also limit training and development opportunities. Ongoing training sessions, team meetings and professional networking opportunities usually take place during the day, which can create a gap between day and night carers. This can lead to a sense of disconnection or marginalization, and pose additional challenges for those seeking to evolve or specialize in their careers.

Despite these drawbacks, for many orderlies the vocation that drives them to choose night duty far outweighs these difficulties. This vocation is fueled by the desire to provide quality care at times when patients are often at their most vulnerable. Working at night means responding to an essential need, looking after those who are ill or in distress when the world is asleep. This mission, imbued with meaning and dedication, gives night work an almost sacred dimension for those who live it as a true vocation.

- **The challenges and responsibilities of the night orderly**
  - **Ensuring continuity of care**

Ensuring continuity of care is a central mission in the nursing auxiliary's work, and takes on an even more critical dimension on night duty. This task involves ensuring that each patient receives uninterrupted care, tailored to his or her specific needs, and that this care is consistent and harmonious, regardless of the time of day or night. It's a daily challenge that demands constant vigilance, rigorous organization, and a genuine commitment to patient well-being.

Continuity of care begins with a smooth and complete handover between the day and night teams. At this precise moment, the caregiver must receive all relevant information on each patient's state of health, the care that has been provided during the day, and any concerns or interventions to be planned during the night. This transfer of information is essential to ensure consistent care, as it enables the night carer to immediately understand priorities, detect warning signs, and anticipate specific patient needs. Good handover ensures that nothing is left to chance, and that every patient continues to receive the attention they need, even in the absence of the daytime teams.

Once the handover has taken place, the night orderly must maintain constant follow-up of patients, ensuring that planned care is carried out accurately and with respect for individual needs. This includes regular monitoring of vital signs, administering prescribed treatments, and adapting care according to changes in the patient's state of health. At night, patients are often more vulnerable, and some signs of deterioration may go unnoticed if attention is not sustained. The caregiver must therefore be vigilant and able to spot any anomalies or subtle changes that may require immediate intervention.

Ensuring continuity of care also requires a high degree of adaptability, as the night is often the scene of unforeseen events and emergencies. A patient who seemed stable may suddenly deteriorate, requiring rapid reassessment and coordinated action with nurses and doctors on call. At such times, the caregiver's ability to remain calm, assess the situation accurately, and act effectively is crucial to the patient's safety and well-being. Every gesture must be measured, every decision taken with an acute awareness of its consequences.

But continuity of care isn't just about managing emergencies or monitoring patients. It also encompasses the human aspect of care, the bond of trust that caregivers forge with patients, even in the darkest hours of the night. For patients, knowing that they are being carefully watched and cared for, even in their sleep, is a key factor in reassurance and comfort. The caregiver's discreet but constant presence embodies this continuity, the invisible thread linking every moment of care, day and night.

Finally, ensuring continuity of care also means preparing the transition to the day shift. At the end of their shift, night carers must pass on all the necessary information on the progress of each patient, the care provided, and any interventions to be planned. This transmission is crucial to ensure that care continues without interruption, and that each patient receives uninterrupted attention. It's a cycle that repeats itself every day, in which every caregiver, whether working day or night, plays an essential role in maintaining the quality and consistency of care.

   ◦   **Managing autonomy and decision-making**
Managing autonomy and decision-making is a fundamental aspect of the nursing auxiliary's work, particularly on night shifts. When the quiet of the night envelops the hospital, shifts are reduced, and situations often have to be managed with fewer resources and less immediate support. In this context, the orderly finds himself on the front line, where his autonomy becomes not only an asset, but a vital necessity to ensure continuity and quality of care.

Autonomy in night work means above all the ability to perform tasks without constant direct supervision. The caregiver must be able to manage the day-to-day care of patients effectively and independently, adhering to established protocols while showing initiative when the situation calls for it. This autonomy manifests itself in the ability to plan and organize care in such a way as to minimize disruption to patients, while ensuring careful monitoring of their state of health. It's not simply a matter of following instructions, but of understanding the overall context of care and acting proactively to prevent complications or respond to changing patient needs.

Decision-making, meanwhile, is closely linked to this autonomy. At night, emergency situations can arise without warning, and the caregiver often has to react quickly, sometimes even before the rest of the night shift is mobilized. Whether managing a respiratory crisis, responding to a patient in distress, or dealing with a sudden change in a patient's condition, the caregiver must be able to make informed decisions in a very short space of time. These decisions rely on their experience, knowledge and clinical judgment, but also on their ability to remain calm under pressure, and to quickly assess the options available.

Another crucial aspect of managing autonomy and decision-making is the caregiver's ability to recognize the limits of his or her role and skills. Working autonomously does not mean working in isolation or refusing to ask for help when necessary. On the contrary, one of the signs of good autonomy management is the ability to correctly assess a situation and know when to alert an on-call nurse or doctor. The caregiver must be able to judge whether a situation can be managed at his or her level, or whether it requires the intervention of professionals with more specialized skills. This lucidity is essential to avoid potential errors and guarantee patient safety.

At night, this autonomy is also put to the test in the management of daily tasks which, although less urgent, are just as important to patients' comfort and well-being. These may include managing hygiene care, repositioning patients to prevent bedsores, or administering simple treatments. Here again, the caregiver must make decisions about the best way to proceed, taking into account each patient's individual needs and adapting care accordingly. This ability to personalize care, to be flexible while respecting protocols, is another key aspect of autonomy.

Autonomy and decision-making on the night shift therefore require a high degree of professional maturity, the ability to anticipate needs and react quickly to unforeseen situations. But they also demand a strong personal ethic, as working autonomously implies increased responsibility. Caregivers must be aware that their decisions and actions have a direct impact on the health and well-being of patients, and this demands a constant commitment to maintaining a high level of competence and professionalism.

○   Collaboration with the multidisciplinary night team

Collaboration with the multidisciplinary night shift team is an essential part of the caregiver's job. In the hospital environment, particularly during the night, effective care depends on the ability of each team member to work together harmoniously, to share crucial information, and to support joint efforts to ensure patient well-being and safety. This collaboration is not simply a professional requirement, it is at the very heart of the night shift operation, where resources are limited and team cohesion becomes a determining factor in the quality of care.

The multi-disciplinary night shift team is generally made up of nursing aides, nurses, doctors on call, security personnel, and sometimes specialized technicians such as radiologists or laboratory technicians. Each of these professionals brings specific expertise to the table, but it's the ability to work together, communicate effectively and support each other that makes the team strong. For the caregiver, this collaboration means first and foremost excellent communication. The transmission of information must be clear, precise and punctual. Every member of the team needs to know what's going on with each patient, what interventions have been carried out, and what actions are still required. This flow of information is crucial to avoiding errors, ensuring smooth continuity of care, and enabling everyone to react quickly in the event of an emergency.

Working in a multi-disciplinary team also demands great adaptability. At night, situations can change rapidly, and priorities often shift as emergencies arise. At such times, the caregiver must be able to adjust to the needs of the moment, taking the initiative while remaining coordinated with other team members. For example, if a patient requires rapid intervention, the caregiver may have to assist the nurse with care, prepare the necessary equipment, or alert the doctor on call. This flexibility is essential if the team is to respond effectively to all situations, even the most unexpected.

The nursing auxiliary also plays a crucial role as a link between patients and the rest of the team. Often spending the most time at the patient's bedside, they are at the forefront of observing clinical signs, detecting changes in health status, and perceiving patients' unexpressed needs. These observations, when shared with the team, enable more responsive and better-adapted care. The caregiver thus becomes a genuine information relay, helping to develop and adjust care plans in real time.

Collaboration with the multidisciplinary team is not limited to emergency situations or direct care. It also includes more subtle aspects, such as the emotional and moral support that team members offer each other. Working at night can be exhausting, and team solidarity is a key factor in maintaining motivation and efficiency. A word of encouragement, a chat about a difficult situation, or simply recognition for a job well done are all small gestures that strengthen team cohesion and create a calmer, more productive working environment.

In addition, working with the multidisciplinary night shift team means understanding and respecting each other's roles and competencies. Caregivers need to know when and how to seek help from nurses, doctors or other specialists, while being aware of their own limitations. This mutual recognition of skills is essential to avoid conflicts, maximize the effectiveness of interventions, and ensure that each patient receives the most appropriate care.

Finally, collaboration within the night shift also prepares the transition to the day shift. At the end of the shift, the information and observations gathered throughout the night must be transmitted clearly and completely to the next shift. This continuity between night and day shifts is fundamental to ensuring that care continues uninterrupted and that patients remain the focus of attention, regardless of staff changes.

Chapter 2
Preparation
Night Service

- **Physical and mental preparation**
  - **Managing the circadian rhythm**

Managing circadian rhythm is an inescapable challenge for caregivers working night shifts. The circadian rhythm, also known as the biological clock, is a natural 24-hour cycle that regulates many physiological processes in our bodies, including sleep, alertness, body temperature and hormone production. This rhythm is synchronized with the light and dark cycles of the environment. However, when we work at night, this cycle is profoundly disrupted, which can have consequences for our physical and mental health. Learning to manage this disruption is essential to maintain well-being and efficiency.

The first challenge in managing the circadian rhythm of night work is to maintain optimal alertness and performance during the hours when the body is naturally programmed to sleep. Between 2 and 4 a.m., for example, drowsiness often peaks, body temperature drops, and production of melatonin - the sleep hormone - increases, making it harder to wake up. To counteract these effects, caregivers need to adopt strategies to stay alert and focused. This can include regular breaks, exposure to bright light (which helps signal the body clock that it's still time to be awake), and avoidance of heavy or carbohydrate-rich meals, which can accentuate drowsiness.

Daytime sleep, which becomes the main rest period for night workers, is another complex facet of circadian rhythm management. Daytime sleep is often of poorer quality than nocturnal sleep. It can be shorter, more fragmented and less deep, partly due to natural light and surrounding noise. To improve the quality of this sleep, the caregiver needs to create an environment conducive to rest: a dark, cool, quiet room, possibly aided by the use of eye masks, earplugs, or white noise machines. Establishing a regular sleep routine, even on days off, can also help stabilize the circadian rhythm and make it easier to fall asleep.

Diet also plays a key role in circadian rhythm management. As the body is accustomed to diurnal eating schedules, eating at night can disrupt digestion and metabolism. It is advisable to eat lightly during the night shift, and to avoid excessively fatty or sugary foods which can cause digestive disorders and affect daytime sleep. It's also important to maintain adequate hydration without abusing caffeine, which, although it helps to stay awake, can disrupt sleep later in the day.

The health impacts of circadian rhythm disruption are another aspect not to be overlooked. Night shift workers are more exposed to certain health risks, such as sleep disorders, cardiovascular disease, diabetes, and mood disorders like depression or anxiety. Stress management is therefore essential. Incorporating relaxation activities, such as meditation, yoga or breathing exercises, can help offset the negative effects of night-time work on the body and mind. In addition, keeping in touch with a doctor for regular follow-up is recommended to monitor the impact of night work on health, and to take the necessary measures in the event of any imbalance.

Last but not least, circadian rhythm management concerns not only the individual, but also those around him or her. Family and social support is crucial to maintaining balance. It's important for family and friends to understand the specific needs of a night shift worker, particularly with regard to rest periods and the need to maintain a calm environment during the day. Maintaining an active social life is also a challenge, but essential to avoid isolation and preserve good mental health.

○   **Impact on health: sleep, diet and well-being**
The health impacts associated with night work are numerous, affecting several essential aspects of life, such as sleep, diet and general well-being. For caregivers, who are often faced with staggered working hours and demanding working conditions, understanding and managing these impacts is crucial to maintaining not only their professional effectiveness, but also their quality of life.

Sleep is undoubtedly the aspect most affected by night shifts. The human body is naturally programmed to sleep at night, when darkness favors the production of melatonin, the hormone that regulates sleep. Working at night disrupts this natural cycle, forcing the body to adapt to an inverted rhythm. This disruption often results in difficulty falling asleep, shallower and more fragmented sleep, and a reduction in total sleep time. Daytime sleep, even under the best conditions, is generally less restorative than nighttime sleep. This sleep deficit can lead to an accumulation of fatigue, reduced alertness and impaired cognitive functions, making work more difficult and increasing the risk of errors. In the long term, this lack of sleep can have serious health consequences, such as an increased risk of cardiovascular disease, diabetes, and mood disorders like depression.

Eating habits are also profoundly affected by night shifts. The body, accustomed to eating during the day, reacts differently when we eat at night. Digestion is slower, and food choices may be less healthy, due to a tendency to eat fast food or sugary snacks to combat fatigue. These unbalanced eating habits can lead to weight gain, digestive disorders, and an increased risk of developing metabolic diseases such as diabetes. What's more, the displacement of meals from the circadian cycle can disrupt blood sugar and lipid regulation, increasing the risk of metabolic disorders. To counteract these effects, it is essential to adopt a diet adapted to night-time working, favoring light meals rich in fiber and protein, and avoiding excess caffeine and sugar.

General well-being, both physical and mental, is also put to the test by night work. Chronic fatigue due to lack of sleep can affect mood, diminish motivation, and provoke a sense of exhaustion that can become overwhelming. The discrepancy with the pace of life in society, where most social and family interactions take place during the day, can lead to feelings of isolation, loneliness and even depression. The difficulty of reconciling work and personal life, exacerbated by night shifts, can also generate stress, affect family relationships, and diminish overall quality of life.

In response to these impacts, it is crucial for caregivers to implement strategies to preserve their well-being. On the sleep front, creating an optimal resting environment is essential: a dark, quiet, cool room can help improve daytime sleep quality. Establishing a regular sleep routine, even on days off, can also help stabilize the sleep cycle. In terms of diet, it's advisable to plan meals so as to maintain balanced nutrition, avoiding heavy meals at night and favoring healthy snacks to maintain energy without compromising digestion.

For mental well-being, maintaining a balance between work and personal life is essential. This can include relaxing activities, sport, and spending quality time with family and friends. Social support is particularly important in combating isolation, as is staying connected with colleagues and sharing experiences of the night shift. Stress management techniques such as meditation, yoga or breathing exercises can also be beneficial in mitigating the negative effects of night work on mental well-being.

- **Specific skills and knowledge to be acquired**
  - **Managing nocturnal emergencies**

Managing nocturnal emergencies is one of the most critical and demanding aspects of night shift work, especially for nursing aides, who are often on the front line when an unexpected situation arises. At night, the quiet, tranquil atmosphere can quickly be turned upside down by the onset of an emergency, requiring rapid reaction, clear judgment and effective coordination with the multidisciplinary team. It's a time when every second counts, and when the ability to manage stress and make decisions under pressure becomes essential.

One of the primary characteristics of night-time emergencies is the need to react with a high degree of autonomy. Indeed, night shifts are generally small, and care assistants often have to take the first initiatives while awaiting the arrival of the nurses or doctors on duty. This means they must be able to quickly assess the seriousness of the situation, stabilize the patient where possible, and initiate the appropriate emergency procedures. This ability to intervene immediately, using acquired knowledge and skills, is crucial to preventing the situation from deteriorating further.

Communication also plays a vital role in managing nocturnal emergencies. At the first sign of an emergency, it is essential that the caregiver quickly and clearly informs the other team members. This communication must be precise, concise and effective, as it enables the necessary resources to be mobilized quickly and ensures optimum coordination between all those involved. Clarity in the transmission of information is all the more important as, at night, there may be fewer responders and they need to divide tasks judiciously to maximize the effectiveness of the response.

Managing nocturnal emergencies also requires rigorous preparation. Although emergencies are, by their very nature, unpredictable, good preparation can make all the difference. This includes thorough knowledge of emergency protocols, familiarity with the location and use of medical equipment, and the ability to perform technical gestures quickly and accurately. Caregivers need to be regularly trained in emergency procedures, take part in simulations, and keep their skills up to date so they're ready to deal with any situation, from cardiopulmonary resuscitation to managing a hemorrhage.

Another crucial aspect is managing stress and emotions. Night-time emergencies can be particularly stressful, due to the nocturnal setting, accumulated fatigue, and the sense of loneliness that can be amplified at night. The caregiver must therefore show great self-control to avoid letting emotions get the better of him or her. This means staying focused on what needs to be done, following protocols rigorously, and demonstrating unfailing composure. The ability to manage stress is a skill that develops with experience, but it can also be supported by relaxation and emotion management techniques, such as controlled breathing or mindfulness.

Finally, managing nocturnal emergencies **doesn**'t stop once the crisis has been resolved. It also includes an important aspect of follow-up and communication with the daytime team. Once an emergency has been managed, it is essential to accurately document the actions taken, the evolution of the patient's condition, and the interventions carried out. This information is crucial to ensure continuity of care, and to enable the day team to take over with full knowledge of the facts. Debriefing with the night team after an emergency is also an important time for analyzing what happened, identifying what went well, and pinpointing areas for improvement. This not only contributes to the continuous improvement of practices, but also strengthens team cohesion and better prepares everyone to deal with future emergencies.

○ **Role in palliative care administration**

The caregiver's role in palliative care is both delicate and profoundly human, requiring a combination of technical skills, empathy and emotional support. Palliative care, which aims to relieve the suffering and improve the quality of life of terminally ill or critically ill patients, places the caregiver at the heart of holistic care, where every gesture and word has a special meaning.

In the administration of palliative care, the caregiver plays a crucial role in ensuring the patient's physical comfort. This is a mission that goes far beyond traditional care, as it involves relieving pain and unpleasant symptoms, such as dyspnea, nausea or anxiety, which often accompany the end of life. The caregiver must be particularly attentive to the patient's needs, adapting care as the patient's condition evolves, and responding proactively to signs of distress. For example, this may involve repositioning the patient to prevent pressure sores, administering gentle hygiene care to avoid discomfort, or adjusting blankets to maintain a comfortable body temperature.

Caregivers are also indispensable in providing emotional support to palliative care patients. At this stage of the disease, patients may experience feelings of fear, anxiety, loneliness and despair. The caregiver, through his or her reassuring presence and active listening, plays a key role in alleviating such psychological suffering. He or she is often the first to perceive the unspoken, to understand the emotions hidden behind a silence or a look, and to offer a soothing word or a comforting gesture. Emotional support is just as important as physical care, helping patients to feel supported, respected and cared for.

In palliative care, the caregiver is also a pillar for families. The end of a loved one's life is a time of great vulnerability, not only for the patient, but also for his or her loved ones, who may feel helpless, overwhelmed by grief, or submerged by uncertainty. The caregiver, by being present alongside the family, guides them through this ordeal. They can explain ongoing care, answer their questions, help them understand what's going on, and comfort them at the same time. Their role is to support them, to offer them a space in which to express their pain, and sometimes simply to be a reassuring presence in these moments of intense emotion.

The administration of palliative care also requires the caregiver to have a strong ability to collaborate with the multidisciplinary team. Palliative care often involves several healthcare professionals, such as nurses, doctors, psychologists and social workers, each bringing specific expertise to offer comprehensive patient care. The caregiver must communicate effectively with these professionals, sharing observations and contributing to the development and adjustment of the care plan according to the patient's needs. This collaboration is essential to ensure that all aspects of the patient's suffering are taken into account and treated appropriately.

In addition, the caregiver must be resilient in the face of the intense emotional burden of palliative care work. Being confronted with suffering, death and bereavement on a daily basis can be taxing, and it's essential that caregivers take care of their own mental health. This may involve seeking support from colleagues, taking part in discussion groups, or finding personal ways of coping with stress and emotions. This resilience is crucial not only to preserving the caregiver's well-being, but also to ensuring that he or she can continue to offer quality, humane and compassionate care.

- **The equipment and tools needed for night duty**
  - **Organizing the care kit**

The organization of the care kit is a fundamental aspect of the caregiver's daily work, particularly on night shifts where efficiency and speed of intervention are crucial. A well-organized care kit not only saves time, but also reduces stress and ensures optimal patient care, especially in emergency situations where every second counts. This organization is not simply a matter of practicality; it reflects meticulous preparation that ensures care can be delivered seamlessly, minimizing interruptions and errors.

The first step in organizing a care kit is to ensure that all the necessary tools and materials are present and in good condition. It's essential to carry out a regular inventory to check that nothing is missing, that instruments are clean and sterilized, and that consumables such as dressings, gloves and compresses are in sufficient quantity. This check should be carried out at the start of each shift to avoid any surprises when dealing with a patient. A well-equipped care kit is a guarantee of peace of mind for the orderly, who knows that he or she has everything he or she needs at hand.

Secondly, the internal organization of the kit is essential to ensure rapid access to the various components. Tools must be arranged

43

logically, according to frequency of use and the order in which they are generally used during care. For example, gloves, which are often the first thing to be used, should be placed on top or in an easily accessible pocket. More specific instruments, such as tweezers, scissors or thermometers, should be stored neatly in separate compartments, to avoid having to search for them when needed. Good organization also means arranging items according to their nature: metal tools together, care products in another compartment, and consumables in a separate area.

Categorizing kit items according to the type of care to be provided is also an effective strategy. For example, it can be useful to group all the materials needed for wound care in a specific compartment, including sterile compresses, saline solution, adhesive dressings and bandages. Similarly, hygiene equipment such as wipes, non-sterile gloves and disinfectants should be kept in a separate compartment. This organization enables the caregiver to find what he or she needs quickly, without having to rummage through the whole kit, which is particularly important in stressful situations or when time is at a premium.

It is also important to ensure that the care kit is adapted to the specific needs of the patients being cared for. For example, if the caregiver works in a department where the majority of patients are in palliative care, the kit should contain, as a priority, materials designed to relieve pain and ensure patient comfort, such as subcutaneous medications, syringes and small-gauge catheters. Similarly, in a pediatric ward, the kit should include child-friendly equipment such as colored dressings and pediatric thermometers. Adapting the care kit to the context allows us to respond more effectively to patient needs and personalize care.

Regular maintenance of the care kit is another essential aspect of its organization. It's not enough to equip it correctly once; it needs to be restocked, cleaned and reorganized regularly to ensure that it remains functional and ready for use. Obsolete products must be removed and replaced, and reusable instruments must be thoroughly disinfected after each use. This regular maintenance is a guarantee of safety, ensuring that the equipment used is always in perfect working order and free from any risk of contamination.

Finally, the organization of the care kit also contributes to the collective efficiency of the care team. A well-organized kit is easy to use by any member of the team, which is crucial in departments where several caregivers may have to intervene on the same patient. Consistency in kit organization within a team means that each caregiver can quickly find the tools they need, even if they're using a kit prepared by a colleague. This standardization is particularly useful in times of emergency, when fast, efficient collaboration between team members is paramount.

◦   **The use of night surveillance tools**

The use of night-time monitoring tools is a crucial aspect of caregivers' work, particularly during the quiet hours of the night, when vigilance must be redoubled to ensure the safety and well-being of patients. These tools, which range from vital signs monitors and alarm systems to more advanced technologies such as motion sensors and infrared cameras, play an essential role in the early detection of anomalies and the prevention of incidents. Their effective use requires not only technical mastery, but also a thorough understanding of their function within the overall framework of night care.

One of the most commonly used tools for nocturnal monitoring is the vital signs monitor, which tracks essential parameters such as heart rate, blood pressure, oxygen saturation and patient respiration in real time. These devices are particularly useful for patients in intensive care or with unstable medical conditions. At night, when the nursing team is reduced, these monitors act as sentinels, immediately alerting the caregiver to any deviation from established norms. The caregiver's ability to interpret this data quickly and respond appropriately is crucial to preventing complications. In the event of an alert, the caregiver must not only check the patient's condition, but also adjust care or inform

45

the on-call nurse or doctor, depending on the severity of the situation.

In addition to vital signs monitors, caregivers often use alarm systems connected to patients' beds, especially for those at risk of falling or suffering from cognitive disorders such as dementia. These alarms are designed to detect the patient's movements when they attempt to get up without assistance, which could lead to serious accidents. When the alarm is triggered, the caregiver must intervene quickly to assist the patient, prevent a fall, and assess whether it is necessary to readjust safety measures, such as reinforcing bed rails or installing anti-fall mattresses on the floor. These tools are particularly valuable at night, when continuous monitoring is more difficult to ensure due to reduced staffing levels.

Motion sensors and infrared cameras are also used in some facilities to monitor patients' movements in specific areas, such as corridors or room exits. These devices make it possible to discreetly track patients' movements without disturbing them, especially those with a tendency to wander due to cognitive or psychological disorders. Caregivers can monitor patients' activity while maintaining their comfort and peace of mind. If a patient moves outside his or her secure zone, the sensors send an alert to the care team, who can then intervene quickly to redirect the patient or accompany him or her to safety. This discreet yet effective surveillance is essential to guarantee patient safety, while respecting their autonomy and dignity.

The use of night-time monitoring tools is not limited to simply detecting anomalies or dangers. It also includes the ability to use these technologies to anticipate patient needs. For example, sensors that monitor patient positions can help prevent bedsores by alerting caregivers when a patient has remained in the same position for too long. In this way, the caregiver can intervene to reposition the patient, improving comfort and reducing the risk of complications linked to immobility. Similarly, sleep monitoring systems, which analyze patients' sleep cycles, can provide invaluable data enabling care to be tailored to respect patients' nocturnal rest while ensuring their safety.

Managing night-time monitoring tools also requires ongoing training and adaptation to technological developments. Caregivers need to be regularly trained in the use of these tools, not only to understand how they work, but also to know how to correctly interpret the data they provide. The rapid evolution of medical technologies means that new devices appear regularly, offering ever more precise and comprehensive monitoring capabilities. Being able to adapt to these new developments and integrate these technologies into care routines is a challenge that caregivers must rise to if they are to continue to provide high-quality care.

Finally, it's important to stress that, despite the effectiveness of night-time monitoring tools, the clinical judgment and direct observation of caregivers remain indispensable. Technologies can offer invaluable support, but they cannot replace the experience, intuition and empathy of a caregiver attentive to the slightest signs of distress or discomfort in his or her patients. Monitoring tools should be seen as decision aids, complementing and enriching the care provided, but they should never diminish the value of human presence with patients, especially during the silent hours of the night.

      ◦   **Tips for maximum efficiency**

Tips for achieving maximum efficiency as a caregiver, particularly on night shift, are essential for navigating an often demanding and unpredictable environment. Efficiency is measured not only by how quickly tasks are completed, but also by the quality of care provided, time management, and the ability to maintain constant vigilance despite the challenges specific to night work. These tips revolve around several key areas: organization, energy management, communication and attention to detail.

Organization is undoubtedly the key to maximizing efficiency. This starts with meticulous preparation before each shift. It's essential to be familiar with each patient's situation, to understand the night's priorities, and to plan tasks according to the patient's state of health and the care to be administered. Having a clear plan of action not only helps to structure the night, but also to manage the unexpected with greater serenity. For example, by prioritizing tasks, the caregiver can ensure that the most critical care is delivered first, while leaving flexibility to respond to emergencies that may arise.

Energy management is another crucial tip for maintaining maximum efficiency throughout the shift. Working at night means fighting against the body's natural rhythm, which is programmed to sleep during this period. To avoid excessive fatigue, it's important to take regular breaks, however short. These moments of rest allow you to recharge your batteries, maintain your vigilance and prevent mistakes due to exhaustion. Good hydration and light but nutritious snacks can also help maintain stable energy levels without causing energy crashes. Avoiding excess caffeine is also recommended, as while it may temporarily stimulate, it can also disrupt sleep once the shift is over, leading to accumulated fatigue over the long term.

Effective communication with the team is also essential to maximize efficiency. At night, when shifts are reduced, coordination and information sharing take on vital importance. Ensuring a clear flow of instructions at the start and end of the shift helps to guarantee continuity of care and avoid misunderstandings. During the shift, maintaining open and regular communication with colleagues helps to distribute tasks evenly and ensure that everyone is aware of developments in patients' conditions. This active collaboration ensures responsiveness and safety, especially in emergencies.

Attention to detail is another key to maximum efficiency. In care, the little things can make a big difference. Taking the time to double-check a prescription, to make sure all equipment is in place before starting a procedure, or to immediately note an observation in the patient's chart, no matter how seemingly trivial, can prevent errors and improve the quality of care. Being meticulous in your work helps avoid backtracking or corrections, which not only saves time, but also boosts the confidence of patients and colleagues.

Another trick is to develop efficient routines. By structuring care in a systematic way, the caregiver can gain in speed and precision. For example, always following the same procedure for preparing care, or organizing the care cart in the same way every night, reduces the time required for reflection and action. Far from being an obstacle to flexibility, these routines create a solid foundation on which the caregiver can build to deal more serenely with the unexpected.

Finally, maximum efficiency also means taking into account your personal well-being. Working efficiently doesn't mean sacrificing your health or your life balance. It's important to take care of yourself, to have a healthy lifestyle, and to ensure that off-duty rest time is truly restorative. This includes good sleep management, a balanced diet, and relaxing activities to unwind after work. A caregiver in good health, both physically and mentally, is better able to cope with the challenges of night work and maintain high efficiency without burning out.

In conclusion, achieving maximum efficiency as a caregiver, especially on night shift, relies on a combination of organization, energy management, communication, and attention to detail. These tricks, if integrated into the work routine, not only save time and reduce stress, but also ensure high-quality care for patients. Efficiency in the care environment is not about doing things quickly, but about doing them well, thoughtfully and in a coordinated way, while taking care of yourself so that you can continue to offer the best of your skills night after night.

Chapter 3
Patient care at night

- **Continuity of care at night**
  ◦ **Handover and transmission of information**

The handover and transmission of information are crucial moments in the day-to-day work of care assistants, particularly on night shifts, where continuity of care depends to a large extent on the quality of this transition. The handover marks the point of connection between two teams, the one ending its shift and the one taking over. It's a time when all information concerning patient condition, care provided, incidents that have occurred, and future actions must be shared clearly, concisely and comprehensively. A well-executed handover ensures that every patient continues to receive consistent, appropriate care, without disruption or confusion.

The handover process generally begins with a meeting between the day and night teams, or vice versa, depending on the direction of the handover. This meeting provides an opportunity to take stock of patients, review priorities and discuss cases requiring special attention. It's a time for dialogue, when outgoing caregivers pass on not only facts and figures, but also their clinical observations, impressions and recommendations based on their experience of the department. Every detail counts, because even a small omission can have a major impact on the quality of care.

The transmission of information during the handover must be structured and systematic. A commonly used method is the "SBAR" (Situation, Background, Assessment, Recommendation) approach, which presents information in an organized, logical way. This method ensures that nothing is forgotten, and that information is presented in such a way as to be quickly understood by the team taking over. For example, for each patient, the caregiver might begin by briefly describing the current situation (Situation), review the relevant history (Background), give his or her assessment of the patient's condition (Assessment), and finally recommend actions to be taken or points of vigilance for the continuation of the service (Recommendation).

Beyond clinical information, handover is also a time when caregivers share more subtle but equally important details, such as patients' emotional reactions, preferences, or difficulties encountered in managing certain aspects of care. This information, which may seem secondary, is essential to providing personalized care tailored to each patient's specific needs. For example, knowing that a patient has been particularly anxious during the night can guide the caregiver taking over to pay particular attention to his or her emotional well-being.

Documentation also plays a central role in handover. Medical records must be kept accurately up to date, recording all relevant interventions, observations and results. These documents serve as a reference not only for the team taking over, but also for the doctors and other healthcare professionals who work with patients. Good documentation avoids misunderstandings, enables the evolution of patients' health to be traced, and facilitates informed decision-making.

However, handover is more than just a transfer of information. It's also a time for mutual support between colleagues. Working the night shift can be stressful, and the handover is an opportunity for caregivers to share their feelings, to debrief on difficult situations, and to ensure that everyone is ready to start or finish their shift in good conditions. This human dimension is essential to maintaining team cohesion and ensuring that caregivers feel supported in their day-to-day work.

Finally, it's crucial that the handover takes place in an environment conducive to concentration and exchange. It must take place in a quiet place, free from distractions, to enable clear and effective communication. The time allotted for the test must be sufficient to ensure that all the information is transmitted completely and without haste. Rushed or sloppy handover can lead to omissions or misunderstandings, compromising continuity and quality of care.

o   **Adapting care to nocturnal pathologies**

Adapting care to nocturnal pathologies is an essential skill for caregivers, especially those who work at night. At night, patients' bodies and minds react differently to illness, and certain pathologies may manifest or worsen at this time, requiring specific attention and adapted care. Understanding these nocturnal particularities enables us to better respond to patients' needs and ensure effective care, even in the quietest hours of the night.

One of the first considerations in adapting night-time care concerns respiratory disorders, such as sleep apnea, asthma or chronic respiratory infections. At night, these pathologies tend to worsen, not least because lying down can exacerbate respiratory difficulties. Caregivers must be particularly vigilant for these signs of respiratory distress. It may be necessary to readjust the patient's position, ensure that breathing aids, such as CPAPs for sleep apnea, are used correctly, and closely monitor for signs of hypoxia. In some cases, it may be necessary to administer specific treatments in response to nocturnal symptoms, always in coordination with the nurse or doctor on duty.

Cardiac pathologies, such as heart failure or rhythm disorders, also require adaptation of night-time care. At night, heart rate and blood pressure can fluctuate, leading to episodes of decompensation in frail patients. It is crucial to monitor vital signs regularly, to ensure that patients take their medication as prescribed, and to be alert to any signs of deterioration, such as increased breathlessness or chest pain. The caregiver must also be ready to intervene in the event of a crisis, immediately alerting the medical team and applying emergency protocols.

Neurological disorders, such as epileptic seizures or confusional syndromes, also present particular challenges at night. Epileptic seizures can occur more frequently during sleep, and it's essential to create a safe environment for at-risk patients, ensuring their beds are secure and eliminating dangerous objects nearby. In the event of a seizure, the caregiver must be able to react quickly, following established protocols to protect the patient and reduce the duration of the seizure. For patients suffering from nocturnal confusion, often exacerbated by the darkness and silence of the night, it may be necessary to adapt the environment by keeping the lights dimmed, maintaining a regular rhythm for care, and reassuring the patient with a soothing presence.

Chronic pain, such as that associated with osteoarthritis or cancer, can also intensify at night, making sleep difficult and disrupting the patient's rest. The caregiver must be attentive to signs of pain, even when they are not clearly expressed, and must be ready to administer the prescribed analgesic treatments, while ensuring their effectiveness. It may also be useful to suggest relaxation techniques or reposition the patient to improve comfort. Managing nocturnal pain is essential not only for the patient's physical well-being, but also to prevent the insomnia and agitation that can ensue.

Digestive disorders, such as gastro-oesophageal reflux or nausea, can also worsen at night, requiring adapted care. Reflux, for example, can be relieved by raising the head of the bed or avoiding heavy meals before bedtime. Caregivers must also be alert to signs of dehydration or gastric discomfort, especially in frail patients or those on medication that can irritate the stomach. In some cases, it may be necessary to administer antacids or other symptomatic treatments in accordance with medical prescriptions.

Finally, psychiatric pathologies such as anxiety, depression or schizophrenia can take on a particular dimension at night. Darkness and silence can exacerbate anxiety or provoke agitation. Caregivers must be highly sensitive in detecting signs of psychological distress, offering emotional support, and, if necessary, administering prescribed sedatives. Communication with the patient is crucial to providing reassurance and a sense of security, which can go a long way to alleviating nocturnal symptoms.

- **Care specific to the night shift**
  ◦ **Monitoring vital signs at night**

Monitoring vital constants at night is an essential task for the caregiver, as it helps to ensure the stability and safety of patients during hours when their vulnerability may be heightened. At night, the human body follows a different rhythm, with natural fluctuations in certain vital constants, such as heart rate, blood pressure, respiration and body temperature. These variations can be accentuated by patients' state of health, the effects of treatments, or the progression of certain pathologies. This is why rigorous and careful monitoring of vital constants is crucial to detect any worrying deviations at an early stage, and to intervene appropriately.

One of the first constants to monitor is heart rate. At night, heart rate naturally tends to slow down due to the predominance of the parasympathetic nervous system, which favors rest and recuperation. However, abnormal variations can occur, particularly in patients with cardiac disorders or those on medication. Excessive bradycardia (abnormal slowing of heart rate) or tachycardia (accelerated heart rate) should immediately alert the caregiver. These signs may indicate a deterioration in the patient's state of health, or an adverse reaction to a treatment. The caregiver must then report these abnormalities to the nurse or doctor on duty and, if necessary, apply stabilization measures pending medical intervention.

Blood pressure is another vital constant to keep a close eye on at night. Like heart rate, blood pressure tends to fall during sleep, a phase when the body relaxes and oxygen and energy requirements decrease. However, abnormal fluctuations in blood pressure, such as marked hypotension or persistent hypertension, can signal complications, particularly in patients with hypertension, kidney disease or dehydration. Hypotension can cause dizziness, falls or malaise in the patient, while uncontrolled hypertension can increase the risk of stroke or heart attack. Caregivers must therefore regularly monitor the blood pressure of at-risk patients, and react promptly to any deviation from normal values.

Monitoring breathing is also crucial, especially in patients with respiratory pathologies such as asthma, chronic obstructive pulmonary disease (COPD), or sleep apnea. At night, breathing can become more shallow, and episodes of apnea or dyspnea (difficulty in breathing) can occur, jeopardizing the patient's oxygenation. Caregivers should be alert to signs of respiratory distress, such as abnormal breath sounds, cyanosis (bluish coloration of the lips or fingers) or unusual agitation. In such cases, it is imperative to check oxygen saturation using a pulse oximeter and, if necessary, administer oxygen or reposition the patient to facilitate breathing.

Body temperature is another vital constant that can show significant variations during the night. A slight drop in temperature is normal during sleep, but significant deviations may indicate an underlying problem, such as infection, hypothermia or septic shock. A nocturnal fever should be particularly monitored, as it may signal the evolution of an infection or an inflammatory reaction. Caregivers should regularly take the temperature of patients at risk, and be ready to implement measures to control it, such as administering antipyretics or adjusting blankets to avoid worsening hypothermia.

Beyond the numbers, monitoring vital signs at night also involves careful observation of patients' behavior and general appearance. Sometimes, subtle signs such as sudden confusion, agitation or lethargy can be the first indicators of decompensation, even before vital constants show significant abnormalities. The caregiver must therefore be vigilant and discerning, combining objective data from measuring devices with a more global clinical assessment to detect any situation at risk.

○ **Managing nocturnal pain**

Managing nocturnal pain is a crucial aspect of caregivers' work, as at night, the perception of pain can be amplified by darkness, silence and the absence of distractions. Patients, already vulnerable because of their condition, may experience an intensification of their painful symptoms, which disrupts their sleep, aggravates their discomfort, and affects their general well-being. For the caregiver, managing nocturnal pain involves more than just administering medication; it implies a holistic and empathetic approach, aimed at relieving the patient's suffering while fostering an environment conducive to rest.

The first step in managing nocturnal pain is to assess the nature and intensity of the pain experienced by the patient. This assessment can be more complex at night, as some patients may be reluctant to express their pain, for fear of disturbing the nursing staff, or out of resignation to their condition. The caregiver must therefore be particularly attentive to non-verbal signs of pain, such as grimaces, agitation, frequent changes of position, or indirect complaints. Gentle, reassuring communication is essential to encourage patients to express their feelings. Using pain assessment tools, such as visual or numerical pain scales, can also help quantify pain and adapt interventions accordingly.

The administration of analgesic medication is often a key component of night-time pain management. Caregivers must ensure that prescribed treatments are administered on time, and that the effects of the medication are closely monitored. This includes administering Tier 1 analgesics, such as paracetamol, through to opioids for more severe pain, in strict compliance with prescribed dosages and intervals. It's also important to monitor the effectiveness of the treatment, checking whether the pain diminishes after administration of the medication, and to note any adverse reactions. If pain persists despite treatment, the caregiver should inform the nurse or doctor on duty to consider adjusting the dosage or introducing another type of treatment.

In addition to medication, the management of nocturnal pain also involves non-pharmacological measures, which can greatly contribute to patient comfort. Repositioning the patient to reduce pressure on painful areas, applying hot or cold compresses, and relaxation techniques such as deep breathing or guided meditation can help alleviate pain. These non-drug interventions are particularly useful for patients who prefer to avoid heavy treatments or who suffer from chronic pain. The caregiver plays a key role in proposing and applying these techniques, tailoring care to the patient's individual preferences and needs.

Creating a soothing environment is also crucial in managing nocturnal pain. The nocturnal environment can accentuate the perception of pain due to silence and isolation. It is therefore important to create a reassuring and comfortable setting, by controlling light and noise, ensuring that the bed is comfortable, and making sure that the patient has access to comforting objects, such as a soft blanket or ergonomic pillow. Attention to these details may seem trivial, but they have a significant impact on the perception of pain and the patient's ability to fall asleep.

Managing nocturnal pain also involves emotional and psychological support. Pain, especially when intense or persistent, can arouse feelings of anxiety, despair or anger in the patient. The caregiver must be present not only to relieve physical pain, but also to soothe these emotions. Listening to the patient, acknowledging his or her suffering, and offering reassuring words can help reduce anxiety and reinforce trust in the care team. This empathic dimension is essential, as it helps create a therapeutic alliance that facilitates comprehensive pain management.

Finally, managing nocturnal pain requires constant vigilance and adaptation of care throughout the night. Pain can fluctuate, and what was effective at one point may no longer be so a few hours later. The caregiver must therefore remain attentive to changes in the patient's condition, and be ready to adjust interventions as pain evolves. This involves regular communication with the rest of the night team, to ensure that all relevant information is shared and that care remains consistent and coordinated.

○ **Managing agitated or anxious patients**

Dealing with agitated or anxious patients is a fundamental aspect of the caregiver's job, especially on night shifts, where the absence of daytime activity, darkness and silence can exacerbate these states. Agitation and anxiety are common responses to a variety of factors, such as pain, fear, confusion or medication side-effects. These states can manifest themselves intensely during the night, requiring a particularly attentive, empathetic and adapted approach to soothe patients and help them regain a sense of security and calm.

The first step in managing agitated or anxious patients is to understand the underlying causes of their condition. Agitation may be a symptom of physical discomfort, such as pain or fever, or an unmet need, such as thirst, hunger or the urge to urinate. Similarly, anxiety can be triggered by psychological factors, such as fear of the unknown, loneliness, or thoughts of illness or death. The caregiver must therefore be sensitive to identifying these triggers, by engaging in dialogue with the patient, observing their behavior, and looking for clues in their environment. This understanding is essential to adapt interventions in a targeted way.

Once possible causes have been identified, it's crucial to create a soothing environment for the patient. At night, darkness and silence can amplify feelings of isolation and anxiety. The caregiver can mitigate these effects by adjusting lighting to create a soft, reassuring ambience, eliminating disruptive noises, and ensuring that the patient feels physically comfortable in bed. Simply rearranging the bed linen, adjusting the room temperature, or repositioning the patient can help reduce agitation. If the patient seems disorientated, reminding them where they are and briefly explaining the situation can also help reduce anxiety.

Communication plays a central role in the care of agitated or anxious patients. The caregiver must use a calm, poised voice, choose simple, reassuring words, and take the time to listen to the patient without judgment. It's important to validate the patient's feelings, acknowledge their discomfort or fear, and offer emotional support. Sometimes, simply staying by the patient's side, holding his or her hand, or speaking softly may be enough to ease his or her mind. In some cases, explaining current procedures or upcoming care, and answering questions, can reduce uncertainty and thus anxiety.

When agitation is marked by more intense physical behavior, such as attempts to get out of bed, remove medical devices, or move uncontrollably, the caregiver must intervene gently but firmly. The aim is to protect the patient from himself, while respecting his autonomy and dignity. For example, it may be necessary to secure the bed with rails, accompany the patient when moving around to prevent falls, or redirect his or her attention to a soothing activity. At such times, it is crucial to avoid any coercive measures that could aggravate the patient's agitation or anxiety.

For patients whose anxiety is linked to cognitive disorders, such as dementia or delusions, redirection and validation techniques can be particularly effective. The caregiver can try to distract the patient by engaging them in conversation on a pleasant topic, proposing a calm activity, or using familiar objects to comfort them. The validation method, which involves entering the patient's reality and responding to rather than correcting his or her emotions, can also help reduce agitation by reinforcing the patient's sense of security.

If necessary, and after assessment by the nurse or doctor on duty, medication can be used to help manage anxiety or agitation, especially if these conditions endanger the patient or seriously disrupt his or her well-being. The administration of sedatives or anxiolytics must always be accompanied by close monitoring to assess the effectiveness of the treatment and adjust the dose if necessary. It is also important to monitor potential side effects and to continue offering emotional support, even after the treatment has been administered.

- **Hygiene and night-time comfort care**
  - **Night-time nursing care**

Night-time nursing care plays a central role in the work of care assistants, as it aims to ensure the comfort, safety and well-being of patients during the quieter hours of the day. At night, patients' needs differ slightly from those during the day, requiring a gentler, more discreet approach to care that respects sleep and rest. Adapting nursing care to these particular conditions not only helps to maintain a high standard of care, but also promotes an environment conducive to recovery.

One of the main aims of night-time nursing care is to minimize sleep disruption while providing the necessary care. Sleep is crucial to a patient's healing and well-being, and any interruption can hinder recovery. For this reason, the caregiver must organize care in such a way as to limit unnecessary awakenings. For example, grouping certain procedures, such as taking vital signs, administering medication and hygiene care, into a single visit helps to reduce the number of awakenings. In addition, it's important to ensure that these procedures are carried out as discreetly as possible: speaking in a low voice, using flashlights or dimmed lights, and avoiding sudden noises all help to preserve the calm needed for patients to rest.

Hygiene care, while essential, must be adapted to the night-time routine to avoid interrupting patients' sleep more than necessary. When it comes to changing pads or repositioning a patient, the caregiver must proceed delicately and efficiently. Using odorless products, wet wipes and absorbent sheets can help make this care more comfortable and less invasive. Similarly, when repositioning to prevent pressure sores, it's important to do so gently to avoid waking the patient completely. If the patient is awake, the caregiver can take advantage of this moment to offer a glass of water, adjust the blankets or check the patient's general comfort, while ensuring that he or she can return to sleep quickly after care.

Managing physiological needs, such as hydration and nutrition, is another aspect of nighttime nursing care. Although patients eat and drink less during the night, some may need light snacks or drinks to avoid dehydration, especially if they are taking diuretic medication or are at risk of undernutrition. This care should be provided in a way that does not disrupt sleep: offering easily digestible food and warm drinks, served in silent containers, can help meet the patient's needs without too many interruptions.

Thermal comfort is also a key element of night-time nursing care. Body temperature tends to drop during sleep, and some patients may wake up feeling cold. The caregiver must therefore ensure that every patient is comfortable, with extra blankets on hand if necessary. On the other hand, it's also important to ensure that the patient doesn't overheat, especially if he or she has a fever. Adjusting the room temperature, checking the air humidity, and adapting bedding are simple but essential gestures to maintain optimal thermal comfort.

Emotional support, although more discreet at night, remains an important aspect of nursing care. For some patients, darkness and silence can accentuate anxiety, loneliness or disorientation, especially those suffering from cognitive disorders or at the end of life. The caregiver must be attentive to these aspects and ready to offer reassuring support, whether by a simple presence, a comforting word, or a gentle gesture. Sometimes, just staying a few minutes with a patient before they fall asleep, or discreetly checking on their well-being during the night, can make all the difference in terms of peace of mind.

Preventing risks such as falls is another crucial aspect of night-time nursing care. At night, the risk of falling can be increased by drowsiness, disorientation or the urge to get up to go to the toilet. The caregiver must anticipate these situations by ensuring that paths are clear, that bedside lights are switched on if necessary, and that the patient knows how to ask for help. Installing bed rails, setting up warning devices, and ensuring that necessities (such as glasses, a glass of water, or the call bell) are within easy reach are simple but effective measures to prevent accidents.

Finally, documentation of overnight care is an important step. It ensures that all interventions have been carried out and that the patient's condition has been continuously monitored. This documentation must be accurate and complete, facilitating handover in the morning and ensuring continuity of care. Observations made during the night can provide valuable information for the treatment and management of patients during the day.

∘ Preventing pressure sores and other complications

The prevention of pressure sores and other complications is a key priority in the care of patients, particularly those who are bedridden or have reduced mobility. Bedsores, also known as pressure sores, are skin lesions that occur as a result of prolonged pressure on an area of the body, often pressure points such as the heels, hips and sacrum. These wounds can develop rapidly and lead to serious complications, such as infection, if they are not treated preventively. For the caregiver, preventing pressure sores and other associated complications requires constant vigilance, in-depth knowledge of risk factors, and a proactive approach to daily care.

The first step in preventing pressure sores is to regularly assess the risks for each individual patient. Some patients are more likely to develop pressure sores because of their state of health, age, nutrition or level of mobility. Patients suffering from chronic diseases, such as diabetes or circulatory disorders, those who are malnourished, or those who are unable to change position without assistance, are particularly at risk. A rigorous assessment enables preventive measures to be put in place, tailored to each individual situation. This assessment must be re-evaluated regularly, as risks may evolve according to the patient's state of health.

One of the most effective ways of preventing pressure sores is to reposition patients regularly to relieve pressure on vulnerable areas. Bedridden patients should be repositioned at least every two hours, and those in wheelchairs should be encouraged to lift themselves regularly to relieve pressure on the buttocks. The caregiver plays a key role in this process, ensuring that position changes are carried out carefully to avoid any rubbing or slipping that could damage the skin. Using gentle mobilization techniques, combining actions with light massage to stimulate blood circulation, can also help prevent pressure sores.

The use of preventive devices, such as anti-bedsore mattresses and cushions, is also crucial. These devices are designed to distribute pressure more evenly and reduce the risk of skin damage. Dynamic air mattresses, for example, alternate pressure under different areas of the body, helping to prevent pressure sores. The caregiver must ensure that these devices are correctly installed and used in accordance with the manufacturer's recommendations. It is also important to regularly check the condition of the devices to ensure that they are working properly and do not need to be replaced or adjusted.

Skin care is another fundamental aspect of pressure sore prevention. The skin of at-risk patients must be inspected regularly for the first signs of redness or irritation, which are the first indicators of excessive pressure. Skin hygiene must be rigorously maintained, with gentle cleansing and appropriate products that do not dry out the skin. The application of barrier creams can also help protect the skin from external aggressions, such as the moisture caused by incontinence. If redness or high-risk areas are detected, the caregiver should immediately report these signs to the nurse for prompt attention.

Nutrition also plays a crucial role in pressure sore prevention. A balanced diet, rich in proteins, vitamins and minerals, is essential to maintain skin health and promote healing. Patients who are malnourished or dehydrated are more likely to develop pressure sores due to the fragility of their skin. The caregiver must therefore be vigilant about the patient's nutritional status, encourage good nutrition, and report any signs of undernutrition or dehydration to the nursing staff for further assessment. In some cases, nutritional supplements may be required to boost the body's natural defenses.

In addition to pressure sores, other complications can arise in bedridden patients or those with reduced mobility, such as urinary tract infections, pulmonary embolism and muscle contractures. Preventing these complications also requires a proactive approach. For example, to prevent urinary tract infections, it's important to ensure proper hydration and intimate hygiene. Patients with urinary catheters need extra monitoring, with regular care to avoid infections. To prevent pulmonary embolism, early and regular mobilization of the lower limbs, even in the form of passive exercise, is essential to stimulate blood circulation and avoid clot formation.

Finally, complication prevention needs to be integrated into a holistic approach to care, which takes into account not only the physical aspects, but also the emotional and psychological well-being of patients. Patients at risk of developing pressure sores or other complications may feel anxious or depressed because of their condition. The caregiver must be attentive to these aspects and offer psychological support, taking the time to listen, reassure and encourage the patient. A reassuring environment and positive communication can play an important role in preventing complications, by strengthening the patient's motivation to participate actively in his or her own care.

- **Helping and accompanying patients and families at night**
    - **Night-time communication: calm and soothing**

Night-time communication, particularly in a care environment, is of particular importance. During the silent, dark hours of the night, the way caregivers interact with patients can have a profound impact on their well-being, sense of security and overall comfort. Calm, soothing communication then becomes not only an essential skill, but also a true art, where every word, every intonation, and every gesture is thought out to reassure and put minds at rest.

At night, patients are often more vulnerable. The silence can amplify their fears, pain and loneliness. In this environment, a soft, calm voice can make all the difference. Caregivers need to be aware of the importance of tone of voice, avoiding any abruptness or loudness that might startle or worry the patient. Speaking in a low voice, with a gentle intonation, helps to maintain a climate of calm. It also helps to avoid disturbing the sleep of other patients, while establishing a personal connection with the one who is awake.

The choice of words is also crucial in nocturnal communication. Patients may feel disoriented or anxious, and it's important to reassure them with well-chosen words. Simple phrases like "I'm here for you", "Everything's fine", or "You can rest easy, I'm watching over you" can have a profoundly soothing effect. The caregiver must also be careful to avoid complex medical terms or lengthy explanations, which could confuse or stress the patient in the middle of the night. The message must be clear, concise and comforting.

The gestures that accompany speech also play an important role. Sometimes, a simple presence is enough to reassure an anxious or agitated patient. A tender gesture, such as placing a hand gently on the patient's arm, readjusting their blanket, or offering them a glass of water, can convey a sense of security and comfort. These simple but caring gestures reinforce the feeling of being cared for, even in the dark of night.

Listening is another essential dimension of nocturnal communication. At night, patients may need to talk about their fears, their pain, or simply to feel heard. The caregiver must be available to listen, without rushing, and let the patient express his or her feelings. This active listening, in which every word the patient says is taken seriously, goes a long way towards calming anxieties. Sometimes, just being able to talk to someone, however briefly, can lighten an emotional burden and allow the patient to relax and get back to sleep.

Non-verbal communication is just as important. Body language, posture and eye contact play a key role in how a patient perceives the caregiver. A warm smile, a sympathetic gaze, or a relaxed attitude can all contribute to creating a reassuring atmosphere. Conversely, a closed posture or shifty gaze can unintentionally convey concern or indifference. The caregiver must therefore be aware of the impact of his or her physical presence, taking care to adopt an open, welcoming posture that puts the patient at ease.

In addition, night-time communication must be adaptable to the specific needs of each patient. Some patients, particularly those with cognitive disorders or dementia, may be more confused or disoriented at night. In these cases, it's important to speak to them clearly and repeatedly, using temporal or spatial cues to help them situate themselves. For example, saying "It's late, it's night and everyone's asleep" can help calm a patient who's wondering where they are or what's going on around them.

Finally, communication between members of the care team during the night must also be calm and measured. Exchanges must be discreet, so as not to disrupt the soothing environment created for patients. Using codes or silent gestures to signal each other, avoiding unnecessary conversations in the vicinity of rooms, and maintaining a climate of tranquillity are practices that enhance patient well-being and team efficiency.

◦ **End-of-life care at night**

Accompanying patients at the end of life at night is a profoundly human and delicate task, in which the caregiver plays an essential role. Silence and darkness at night bring a special dimension to the care of patients at the end of life, making every gesture, every word and every presence even more meaningful. It's a time when care is no longer limited to the physical, but encompasses the whole being, in its emotional, psychological and spiritual dimensions.

The first reality of end-of-life care at night is the importance of presence. Simply being there, by the patient's side, can bring immense comfort. In those hours when the world seems to be asleep, the presence of a caring, attentive person can soothe fears, ease loneliness and offer a sense of security. The caregiver becomes a reassuring figure, a landmark in the darkness, bringing human warmth where the patient might feel alone in the face of impending doom. Sometimes, this presence needs no words: the simple act of holding the patient's hand, smiling gently, or remaining silently at his or her side is enough to bring profound comfort.

Communication, even when reduced to gestures or whispers, takes on a special significance in this context. Words must be chosen with care, to offer comfort without raising false hopes. Simple, soothing phrases like "I'm here for you", "You're not alone", or "All is at peace" can help ease the patient's mind. For those who can still express their thoughts, it's essential to listen attentively, without judgment or haste. Letting patients talk about their fears, regrets or memories can be a way of accompanying them in a final, calming dialogue. When words fail, shared silence can become an equally powerful form of communication.

Providing end-of-life care at night also means paying even greater attention to the patient's physical needs. Pain management, for example, is a top priority. The caregiver must ensure that the patient is not in pain, by monitoring signs of pain and carefully administering prescribed medication. Beyond physical pain, the patient's general comfort is paramount: adjusting blankets, repositioning the body to avoid pressure points, moistening the lips, or simply checking that the room temperature is comfortable. These small gestures, often imperceptible but imbued with solicitude, contribute to creating an atmosphere of gentleness and well-being.

Caregivers must also be alert to signs of anguish or respiratory distress that may arise at the end of life. These situations require immediate intervention, but always with calm and gentleness, so as not to aggravate the patient's discomfort. This may involve adjusting oxygen administration, readjusting the patient's position to facilitate breathing, or simply offering reassuring words to alleviate anguish. In these critical moments, every action must be marked by compassion and respect for the patient's dignity.

At night, end-of-life care also extends to the patient's loved ones, if they are present. The night can exacerbate their pain, fatigue and sense of helplessness. The caregiver must be there for them too, offering them discreet but constant support. Sometimes this simply means listening to their concerns, explaining what's happening in simple words, or offering them a cup of coffee to comfort them. It can also mean encouraging them to take a moment's rest, reassuring them that the patient is in good hands. This support for loved ones is essential, as it helps ease their emotional burden and helps them to live through these moments as serenely as possible.

There is also a spiritual dimension to end-of-life care, which can become more pronounced at night. For some patients, the end of life is a time when profound questions about life, death and the afterlife emerge. The caregiver must be ready to accompany the patient in these reflections, without imposing his or her own beliefs, but respecting those of the patient. This may involve praying with the patient if desired, calling in a chaplain or spiritual representative, or simply listening to the patient's thoughts. Respecting the patient's spiritual dimension means recognizing their need to find meaning and peace in their final moments.

◦ **Psychological support for families at night**

Psychological support for families during the night is an essential aspect of the caregivers' work, particularly at times of great vulnerability when the darkness of night seems to accentuate anxieties and worries. When families look after their hospitalized loved ones during the night, they are often faced with a heavy burden of loneliness, fatigue and deep uncertainty about their loved one's state of health. The caregiver, in this context, plays a crucial role in providing not only medical care, but also the emotional support that is indispensable in helping families through these difficult hours.

The first form of support that caregivers can offer families at night is their simple presence. When a loved one is seriously ill or at the end of life, the night can be a particularly anxious time for families. The silence of the corridors, the slowdown in hospital activities, and the perception of isolation can amplify fears and negative thoughts. The caregiver's attentive, reassuring presence can help alleviate these feelings. Even without speaking, the knowledge that someone competent and caring is nearby can bring great comfort. A smile, a look of understanding, or a discreet presence beside them can be enough to give them a sense of security.

Dialogue is also a powerful tool in the psychological support of families. At night, families may need to talk, to express their fears and doubts, or simply to understand what is going on. The caregiver must be a good listener, ready to answer questions with patience and empathy. It's important to provide clear, reassuring information, while being honest about the situation. Explaining what care is being given, what treatments are being administered, or simply how the patient's condition is progressing, can help to ease worries and give a degree of control to families, who often feel helpless in the face of illness.

Caregivers must also be attentive to the emotional fatigue of families. At night, this fatigue can become overwhelming, exacerbated by lack of sleep and accumulated stress. The caregiver can suggest simple solutions to help families take care of themselves, such as taking a break, resting in an adjoining room, or drinking a glass of water. Sometimes a small gesture of kindness, such as bringing an extra blanket or offering a hot drink, can make a big difference. These gestures show families that they are not alone in their ordeal, and that they have the right to take care of themselves, even at such an intense time.

During the night, psychological support also involves recognizing families' emotions. The caregiver must be able to understand and validate these emotions, whether they be fear, sadness, anger or despair. Simply saying "I understand it's difficult" or "It's normal to feel this way" can help families feel understood and supported. It's also important to respect everyone's emotional rhythm, allowing families to experience their emotions without judging them or rushing them into a state of acceptance or calm. The role of the caregiver is to accompany, not force, by providing a safe space where families can express their feelings.

Sometimes, psychological support means accepting that you don't have all the answers. At night, when doctors are not always immediately available, it can be difficult for the caregiver to answer all the family's questions. At such times, honesty and transparency are essential. Saying "I don't know, but I'll try to find an answer for you" or "I'll pass the message on to the medical team as soon as possible" can reassure families that their concerns are being taken seriously. The important thing is to show a willingness to support and do everything possible to get answers, while maintaining open and respectful communication.

Psychological support for families during the night also extends to assistance at critical moments, such as when a patient is nearing the end of life. These moments are often the most emotionally charged, and families can feel totally overwhelmed. The caregiver can offer invaluable support by being present at their side, gently guiding them through the stages of care, and helping them cope with the inevitable. This can include helping

72

them say goodbye to their loved one, supporting them physically and emotionally, and offering them a space to express their pain.

Chapter 4
Managing night-time emergencies

- **Identify and respond to emergency situations**

  ○ **Clinical signs to watch for at night**

The clinical signs to watch out for in an emergency at night are of paramount importance to the caregiver, as they can signal a rapid deterioration in a patient's state of health. At night, when staffing levels are low and it's quiet, these signs can go unnoticed if they are not given careful attention. Yet rigorous monitoring and immediate response can make the difference between effective intervention and serious complications. Identifying these warning signs early on enables us to take the necessary action, while ensuring the safety and well-being of our patients.

One of the first clinical signs to watch out for is respiratory distress. Changes in breathing frequency or quality, such as rapid breathing (tachypnea), irregular breathing, or pauses in breathing (apnea), should immediately alert the caregiver. Unusual breathing sounds, such as rales, wheezes or snoring, are also indicators that something is wrong. These symptoms can signal conditions such as respiratory failure, an exacerbation of chronic obstructive pulmonary disease (COPD), or an asthma attack. In such cases, the caregiver should immediately check the patient's oxygen saturation, reposition the patient to facilitate breathing, and alert the nurse or doctor on duty for further assessment and prompt management.

Another critical sign to watch out for is sudden, intense pain, especially if it's located in the chest, abdomen or head. Chest pain, for example, can be a sign of myocardial infarction or pulmonary embolism, situations that require emergency intervention. Sharp abdominal pain could indicate intestinal perforation, appendicitis or a pancreatitis attack, while sudden head pain could signal a stroke or cerebral hemorrhage. The caregiver must quickly assess the intensity of the pain, its evolution, and associated signs such as pallor, sweating, or confusion, and immediately alert emergency medical services.

76

Altered consciousness is also a major clinical sign to watch out for. A patient who suddenly becomes confused, disoriented or drowsy, or shows a loss of consciousness, should be considered urgently. These signs can be linked to a variety of causes, such as severe hypoglycemia, cerebral hemorrhage, drug intoxication or sepsis. The caregiver should assess the patient's responsiveness by asking simple questions, evaluating his or her ability to move around or follow instructions, and noting any changes from his or her usual state of wakefulness. Rapidly taking vital vitals, particularly blood sugar and blood pressure, is essential to directing first aid until reinforcements arrive.

Cardiovascular abnormalities should also be carefully monitored. Sudden tachycardia, severe bradycardia, or arrhythmias can indicate serious heart problems, such as decompensated heart failure, infarction, or atrial fibrillation. Signs such as palpitations, chest pain, shortness of breath or extreme fatigue should immediately alert the caregiver. Continuous monitoring of heart rhythm, combined with emergency medical care, is crucial to prevent serious complications.

Signs of shock, whether hypovolemic, septic or anaphylactic, are another category of warning signs to watch out for. Shock often manifests itself as marked hypotension, tachycardia, cold clammy skin, mottling and altered consciousness. In the presence of these symptoms, the caregiver must react quickly by monitoring vital signs, keeping the patient in a supine position with legs elevated, and administering oxygen if necessary. Coordination with the medical team for rapid intervention is essential to stabilize the patient's condition.

Another sign not to be overlooked is the onset of high fever, especially if accompanied by chills, profuse sweating, confusion or stiff neck. These symptoms may indicate a severe infection, such as meningitis, septicemia or systemic infection, which requires immediate treatment. The caregiver should take the patient's temperature, note any associated symptoms, and alert the nurse or doctor for appropriate assessment and treatment.

Finally, acute gastrointestinal disturbances, such as persistent vomiting, severe diarrhea, or absence of stool and gas in a postoperative patient, may indicate serious complications such as intestinal obstruction, peritonitis or severe dehydration. The caregiver should monitor these symptoms, ensure that the patient is hydrated as much as possible, and promptly alert the medical team for further assessment.

○ Managing cardio-respiratory emergencies

The management of cardio-respiratory emergencies is a vitally important task for the nursing auxiliary, particularly on night shifts where speed and efficiency are crucial. Cardio-respiratory emergencies, which include situations such as cardiac arrest, myocardial infarction, pulmonary embolism and acute respiratory distress, require constant vigilance and immediate responsiveness. For the caregiver, this means not only recognizing the signs of such an emergency, but also knowing how to intervene rapidly to stabilize the patient while awaiting the arrival of the medical team.

The first step in managing cardio-respiratory emergencies is rapid recognition of the warning signs. A patient presenting with severe chest pain, dyspnea (difficulty breathing), cyanosis (bluish discoloration of the lips or extremities), or loss of consciousness should immediately be considered a cardio-respiratory emergency. Chest pain, often described as oppression or a feeling of weight on the chest, is particularly indicative of a myocardial infarction. In these situations, it's vital not to minimize symptoms and to act quickly.

When cardiac arrest is suspected, the first reflex should be to check the patient's consciousness and breathing. If the patient is unresponsive and not breathing normally, the caregiver must immediately call for help, activate the emergency protocol, and begin cardiopulmonary resuscitation (CPR). CPR consists of performing chest compressions at a sustained rate, combined with air insufflations if the caregiver is trained in this technique, to maintain blood circulation and oxygenation of vital organs. The speed with which CPR is initiated is crucial to increasing the patient's chances of survival. In many institutions, the use of an automatic external defibrillator (AED) is also recommended. This easy-to-use device analyzes the heart's rhythm and delivers an electric shock if necessary in an attempt to restore a normal cardiac rhythm.

In the event of acute respiratory distress, the caregiver must also intervene without delay. If a patient shows signs of respiratory insufficiency, such as rapid, shallow or labored breathing, or is in obvious distress with low oxygen saturation, it is imperative to help him/her into a semi-seated position to facilitate breathing. Oxygen administration, if available and prescribed, must be initiated immediately. In these moments, every second counts, and it is essential to keep the airway clear, while carefully monitoring the evolution of the situation. The caregiver must stay with the patient, monitor vital signs, and be ready to adjust oxygen therapy as required.

When a pulmonary embolism is suspected, usually due to the sudden onset of acute chest pain, dyspnea and sometimes symptoms of shock, the caregiver must immediately alert the medical team. Management of this emergency involves keeping the patient at rest, administering oxygen and monitoring vital signs, while awaiting the arrival of doctors who can confirm the diagnosis and initiate the appropriate treatment. It's crucial to remain calm and act methodically, as anxiety can worsen the situation for the patient.

Communication with the medical team and other nursing staff is another fundamental aspect of managing cardio-respiratory emergencies. At the first sign of such an emergency, the caregiver must immediately report the situation and request assistance, while providing clear and precise information on the symptoms observed, the patient's condition, and the interventions already in place. This rapid, effective communication helps to coordinate the team's efforts and ensure that all necessary resources are mobilized.

Once the emergency has been stabilized or is being managed, it is essential to accurately document the events, the interventions carried out, and the patient's response to treatment. This documentation is crucial for the patient's follow-up and for the medical team that will take over from him/her. It also enables subsequent interventions to be analyzed, so that lessons can be learned and management protocols improved.

Finally, after such an intervention, it's important for the caregiver to take a moment to assess his or her own reaction to the event. Cardiopulmonary emergencies are extremely stressful situations, and it's normal to feel anxious or stressed after such an experience. Discussing the event with colleagues, participating in a debriefing, or simply taking a moment to breathe and refocus is essential to maintaining one's own psychological well-being and being prepared for future emergencies.

- **Collaboration with the night shift**
  - **Division of tasks in an emergency**

The division of tasks in the event of an emergency is an essential component of effective management of critical situations in the hospital environment, particularly on night shifts where human resources may be limited. When an emergency arises, clear organization and harmonious coordination of the care team's efforts are crucial to ensuring a rapid, effective response tailored to the seriousness of the situation. The caregiver, often on the front line, plays a key role in this division of labor, not only by actively participating in interventions, but also by helping to structure and direct the team's actions.

At the first sign of an emergency, whether cardiac arrest, respiratory distress or other critical situation, the priority is to remain calm and immediately sound the alarm. This alert must be clear and concise, informing the entire care team of the nature of the emergency and the patient's location. The caregiver must ensure that the correct emergency protocols are activated, by pressing emergency call devices and communicating directly with available team members.

Once the alarm has been sounded, tasks need to be allocated quickly, according to each person's skills and roles. If they are the first on the scene, orderlies can initiate first aid measures such as cardiopulmonary resuscitation (CPR) in the event of cardiac arrest, or oxygen administration in the event of respiratory distress. These first actions are crucial to stabilizing the patient and buying time until more specialized help arrives.

The nurse, often responsible for immediate medical supervision, will take over to assess the patient's condition, administer medication if necessary, and coordinate more complex care. Meanwhile, the orderly may be entrusted with other essential tasks, such as preparing medical equipment, bringing in defibrillators, or assisting the nurse with more technical procedures. Each member of the team needs to know exactly what he or she has to do, to avoid any confusion or loss of time that could compromise patient care.

The distribution of tasks in an emergency also requires continuous, effective communication between team members. The caregiver must ensure that everyone is kept informed of developments in the situation, and that current needs are clearly expressed. For example, if it is necessary to change tasks or request additional reinforcements, this must be communicated immediately and clearly. This fluidity in communication enables the team to adapt quickly to changes in the patient's condition, and ensures that every action is coordinated.

As part of the division of labor, it is also important to designate a coordinator or leader to direct operations. This role is usually played by the nurse or doctor supervising the operation. The coordinator ensures that tasks are correctly assigned, that actions are carried out in the right order, and that priorities are respected. By following the coordinator's instructions, the caregiver helps to maintain the order and efficiency of the intervention.

Alongside direct intervention, certain support tasks are just as crucial in an emergency. For example, the caregiver may be responsible for managing the immediate environment, ensuring that the space around the patient is clear, that medical devices are functional, and that necessary medication is within easy reach. He or she may also be responsible for reassuring other patients, or communicating with the families present, calmly explaining what's happening and keeping them informed of developments.

After the immediate management of the emergency, the division of tasks also includes follow-up and documentation. The orderly may be responsible for recording the interventions carried out, the vital signs taken, and the patient's response to the treatments administered. This documentation is essential for medical follow-up and post-emergency assessment. In addition, it may be necessary to reorganize regular tasks to compensate for the time and resources mobilized by the emergency, ensuring that the routine care of other patients is not neglected.

Finally, once the emergency has been resolved, a debriefing is often useful to review task allocation and identify strengths as well as areas requiring improvement. By taking part in this debriefing, the orderly helps to refine emergency protocols and strengthen team cohesion for future situations.

◦ **Communication with doctors on call and emergency services**

Communication with doctors on duty and emergency services is an essential part of the nursing auxiliary's role, particularly on night shifts when medical presence may be reduced and emergency situations require exemplary responsiveness. Effective communication is crucial to ensuring that patients are cared for quickly and appropriately, guaranteeing that essential information is conveyed accurately, clearly and in the shortest possible time.

When an emergency situation arises, the caregiver is often the first to assess the patient's condition and detect signs of deterioration. The ability to recognize these signs quickly and alert the doctor on duty or the emergency services is paramount. Initial communication should be concise but comprehensive, providing key information such as the patient's identity, observed symptoms, relevant vital signs, and any interventions already in place. For example, in the case of respiratory distress, the orderly might communicate: "Patient in room 202, Mr. Dupont, 72 years old, presents with severe dyspnea, saturation 82% despite oxygen therapy at 5 L/min, labored breathing. CPR in progress."

This first communication is often decisive, as it allows the doctor on call or the emergency team to prepare themselves mentally and materially for the operation. It is essential that the caregiver remains factual and avoids overloading the doctor with irrelevant details in this first contact. The aim is to convey a clear and immediate picture of the situation, so that healthcare professionals can assess the severity and plan the next steps.

Once the on-call doctor or emergency services have arrived, communication must continue in a fluid, structured manner. The caregiver must be ready to provide additional information, answer questions, and clarify any elements that may be ambiguous. Accuracy in transmitting data is crucial to avoid misunderstandings that could delay or complicate the procedure. For example, if the patient has a particular medical history, such as a drug allergy or pre-existing heart condition, this should be mentioned as soon as possible.

Active listening is also an essential skill in this context. The caregiver must be attentive to instructions given by the doctor or emergency services, implementing them quickly and accurately. This may include tasks such as preparing equipment, administering medication, taking additional vital signs, or assisting with emergency medical procedures. Communication is not a one-way street: it's important that the caregiver feels able to ask questions or seek clarification if necessary, to ensure that the care provided is accurate and appropriate.

In addition, communication with on-call doctors and emergency services must be calm and professional, even in situations of intense stress. The ability to maintain a calm demeanor not only helps to facilitate cooperation between different team members, but also contributes to reassuring patients and their families, who may witness the intervention. A calm tone and controlled demeanor reinforce confidence and effective communication.

Once the emergency is under control, communication doesn't stop there. It is essential to review with the doctor the patient's condition, the care administered, and the next steps. The caregiver must ensure that all actions are properly documented in the patient's medical record, including the interventions of the on-call doctor and emergency services, as well as the clinical evolution observed. This documentation is crucial to the patient's follow-up by day teams and to the continuity of care.

Finally, after the intervention, a feedback or debriefing session with the doctor on duty and the team can be beneficial for all those involved. This helps to review what went well, identify areas for improvement, and strengthen coordination for future interventions. The caregiver can bring valuable perspectives to these discussions, sharing first-hand experience of the situation and offering suggestions for improving communication protocols.

- **Managing stress and emotions in emergency situations**
  - ○ **Self-control in an emergency**

Self-control in an emergency is an indispensable quality for healthcare assistants, especially when critical situations arise unexpectedly and require an immediate and effective response. In the hospital environment, where every second can mean the difference between life and death, the ability to remain calm, focused and rational under pressure is not only an asset, but a necessity. This self-control enables the orderly to manage emergency situations with the mental clarity and precision of execution that are crucial to ensuring the safety and well-being of patients.

In the first few seconds of an emergency, shock or panic could easily overwhelm anyone. However, the caregiver must immediately channel his or her emotions to focus on the essentials: rapidly assessing the situation, identifying critical clinical signs, and initiating the first interventions. Self-control enables the caregiver to filter out the noise, distractions and agitation that can surround an emergency situation, to focus solely on the actions to be taken. It is this ability to ignore the stressful environment that enables the caregiver to remember emergency protocols, apply life-saving gestures, and make informed decisions in an instant.

A key aspect of self-control is managing physiological stress. Faced with an emergency, the body naturally reacts with a surge of adrenaline, which can lead to palpitations, accelerated breathing, or even tremors. The caregiver, aware of these reactions, must know how to control them by using deep breathing techniques, maintaining a stable breathing rhythm, and concentrating on rational thoughts. This keeps you physically calm, preserves the energy you need for the procedure, and avoids errors caused by excessive haste.

Self-control is also expressed in communication with the care team and patients. During an emergency, it's easy to give in to the temptation to speak quickly or give jerky orders. However, clear, poised, structured communication is essential to coordinate the team's efforts and avoid misunderstandings. The caregiver must speak confidently, without raising his or her voice unnecessarily, giving precise instructions and ensuring that everyone understands their role. This calm attitude inspires confidence in other team members, promotes better collaboration, and helps maintain an orderly working atmosphere, even at the most tense moments.

Moreover, self-control implies a certain ability to manage one's emotions, especially in the face of situations that can be emotionally taxing, such as the death of a patient or the obvious anguish of loved ones. The caregiver must be able to put aside his or her own feelings to remain fully focused on the task in hand. This does not mean being insensitive, but rather being able to defer the expression of one's emotions so as not to interfere with the patient's care. After the emergency, it is essential to take the time to process these emotions, either through discussions with colleagues, or through moments of personal reflection, so as not to accumulate stress or emotional fatigue.

Last but not least, self-control is the key to sound decision-making. In an emergency situation, many variables have to be taken into account in a very short space of time. The caregiver must be able to prioritize actions, to judge which interventions are the most urgent and appropriate, and not let himself be overwhelmed by the magnitude of the situation. This lucidity, nurtured by solid training and acquired experience, is essential to avoid impulsive or poorly coordinated actions that could worsen the patient's condition.

However, it's important to recognize that self-control doesn't mean the total absence of stress or emotion. It's natural, even for the most experienced professionals, to feel a certain amount of tension in the face of urgency. The difference lies in the way this stress is managed. The caregiver who masters his or her reactions uses this energy to stay focused and efficient, transforming stress into a driving force rather than an obstacle.

After an emergency, self-control also means knowing how to release the pressure. Once the emergency is over, it's essential to take a moment to decompress, to check on one's own emotional state, and to share with colleagues what happened. Not only does this help to prepare you for future interventions, it also helps to maintain mental and emotional balance over the long term, thus avoiding the risk of burn-out.

○ **Debriefing after a critical situation**

Debriefing after a critical situation is an essential part of the care process, particularly for nursing aides who are on the front line during such events. This process not only allows us to look back on the events that took place, but also to consolidate the collective experience, identify the strengths and weaknesses of the intervention, and reinforce team cohesion. Debriefing is a key step in learning from critical situations, improving future practices, and ensuring the psychological well-being of the healthcare professionals involved.

When a critical situation arises, adrenalin, stress and the urgency of the moment can mask certain details or create different perceptions among team members. Debriefing offers a space for reflection, where everyone can express their point of view, share their feelings, and analyze the facts with the necessary distance. By looking back on the experience, we can reconstruct the sequence of events in a structured way, and identify what went well and what could have been improved.

Debriefing generally begins with a round-table discussion, during which each team member is invited to share his or her feelings and perspective on the situation. The orderly, in particular, can provide valuable information on initial observations, actions taken before the rest of the team arrives, and how he or she experienced the intervention. This sharing of information helps to create a global vision of the situation, taking into account the different stages of the intervention, the decisions made, and the actions taken.

An essential part of debriefing is identifying the strengths of the intervention. This involves highlighting what worked well, whether it was speed of execution, effective communication between team members, or the application of protocols. Recognizing these positive aspects is crucial to boosting caregivers' self-confidence and consolidating practices that have proved effective. It also contributes to valuing the work accomplished and maintaining a positive dynamic within the team.

At the same time, the debriefing must also address areas for improvement. The aim is to identify the difficulties encountered, any mistakes made, or moments when coordination may have been less fluid. It's not a time for personal criticism, but an opportunity for collective reflection to understand what didn't work as planned, and to consider solutions for the future. For example, if communication problems have slowed down the intervention, the debriefing provides an opportunity to discuss ways of improving communication in future critical situations.

Debriefing also has an emotional dimension. Critical situations can be psychologically challenging, and it's important to acknowledge the emotions that everyone may have felt. Debriefing offers a safe space to express these emotions, whether stress, frustration or sadness. This expression helps to release some of the accumulated tension, to feel supported by colleagues, and to strengthen the team's resilience in the face of the challenges encountered. For the caregiver, who may have experienced moments of great emotional intensity, this stage is crucial in preventing burnout and in promoting a return to equilibrium after the crisis.

Debriefing is not just about analyzing what happened, but also about taking concrete action. The lessons learned from the critical situation must be integrated into the team's daily practices. This may include adjustments to protocols, training sessions to reinforce certain skills, or changes to the organization of work to improve responsiveness to emergencies. Debriefing is thus a lever for continuous improvement, enabling the team to become stronger and more efficient with each new experience.

Finally, debriefing strengthens team cohesion. By sharing successes and difficulties, team members come closer together, develop a better understanding of each other and strengthen their mutual trust. This cohesion is essential for dealing with future critical situations, as it creates a working environment where everyone feels supported, respected and valued.

Chapter 5
La Vie
Night shift

- **Interprofessional relations on the night shift**
  - **Working in tandem with the night nurse**

Working in pairs with the night nurse is a fundamental component of the efficient operation of care services, especially during the night hours when shifts are small and each member of staff plays a crucial role. This partnership is based on complementary skills, fluid communication and mutual trust, which are essential for ensuring continuity of care, managing emergency situations, and responding to patients' needs with speed and precision.

Working in tandem with the night nurse creates a synergy, where the specific skills of each are put to good use to offer comprehensive, high-quality care. The nursing auxiliary, with its in-depth knowledge of basic care, hygiene and patient comfort, plays a central role in observing clinical signs, managing daily needs and maintaining patient well-being. Nurses, for their part, contribute their expertise in more technical care, administering treatments, and managing complex situations. Together, they form a strong team capable of responding to a wide range of situations, from routine care management to emergency response.

Communication is one of the cornerstones of working in pairs. Clear, direct and continuous communication between the orderly and the nurse is essential to ensure that each has a complete picture of the patient's condition and the interventions required. Right from the start of the shift, a structured exchange of information enables each patient's situation to be reviewed, the night's priorities to be discussed, and tasks to be allocated according to skills and needs. Throughout the night, this communication continues seamlessly, with regular updates on patient progress, care provided, and any new observations. This constant interaction ensures that nothing is left to chance and that care is optimally coordinated.

Working in pairs with the night nurse also requires great flexibility and the ability to adapt to changing patient needs. At night, situations can change rapidly, and it's crucial that the orderly and nurse can adjust their approach to suit the circumstances. For example, if an emergency arises, the nurse may need to concentrate on the medical aspects of care, while the orderly provides logistical support, prepares the necessary equipment, and ensures the comfort of other patients to avoid unnecessary disruption. This dynamic division of roles maximizes the efficiency of the intervention and ensures that all aspects of care are covered.

The pairing formed by the care assistant and the night nurse is also based on mutual trust. This trust is built up over time, through shared experience and mutual knowledge of each other's skills. The nurse must be able to rely on the caregiver to detect the first signs of deterioration in a patient, to carry out care rigorously, and to provide unfailing support when needed. In turn, the caregiver must trust the nurse to make appropriate clinical decisions, to provide clear direction, and to recognize the importance of his or her role in the team. This mutual trust is a key element in strengthening the pair's cohesion and enabling them to work in harmony, even in the most stressful situations.

Working side-by-side with the night nurse is also a source of continuous learning. Working side by side with a nurse enables the caregiver to develop his or her skills, acquire new knowledge, and deepen his or her understanding of the more technical aspects of care. The nurse, in turn, benefits from the orderly's expertise in basic care and patient observation. This exchange of knowledge and experience contributes not only to the improvement of individual practices, but also to the overall enrichment of the care team.

Finally, working in pairs with the night nurse fosters the creation of a professional relationship based on respect and collaboration. The challenges of the night, with its moments of calm but also its unforeseen emergencies, create an environment where solidarity and mutual support are essential. This working relationship, based on mutual assistance and recognition of each other's skills, creates a framework conducive to both the quality of care and the well-being of healthcare professionals.

◦ **Night shift cohesion and support**

Cohesion and support within the night team are essential to ensure smooth and efficient operation in an often demanding and sometimes isolated environment. Working at night presents unique challenges, such as increased fatigue, feelings of isolation from daytime teams, and managing emergency situations with limited resources. In this context, solidarity between team members becomes not only a factor of well-being for each caregiver, but also a guarantee of quality patient care.

Night team cohesion is built above all on a foundation of clear, open communication. Unlike day teams, where interactions with different professionals and departments are more frequent, the night team often operates on a skeleton staff, making internal communication all the more crucial. It's essential that every team member feels free to share observations, concerns and suggestions without fear of judgment. Fluid communication not only ensures that everyone is on the same wavelength, but also prevents misunderstandings and anticipates problems before they escalate. This transparency builds trust between team members and ensures that care is optimally coordinated.

Mutual support is another pillar of night shift cohesion. Working in the dark, with a reversed circadian rhythm, can lead to moments of intense fatigue and low morale. At such times, the support of colleagues becomes indispensable. It can be as simple as offering to cover a colleague for a break, or as attentive listening when a team member is going through a difficult period. This support is not limited to the professional aspects, but also encompasses emotional well-being. Knowing that colleagues can be counted on for help, or to share a comforting word, creates a working environment where everyone feels valued and understood.

Solidarity within the night shift is also reflected in the fair distribution of tasks. Given the small number of staff, it's crucial that responsibilities are shared in a balanced way, taking into account everyone's skills and strengths. A fair distribution of tasks prevents certain team members from feeling overloaded or neglected, and enables everyone to contribute fully to the smooth running of the night. This fairness in the workload reinforces the feeling of belonging to a close-knit team, where every contribution is recognized and appreciated.

Night shift work also requires great flexibility and the ability to adapt quickly to unforeseen circumstances. Emergencies can arise at any time, and it's essential that every team member is ready to adjust priorities to meet patients' immediate needs. This flexibility is facilitated by team cohesion: when a critical situation arises, team members must be able to coordinate quickly, divide tasks efficiently and act in concert. Mutual knowledge of each other's skills and strengths enables roles to be better allocated according to the needs of the moment, and ensures a rapid and appropriate response.

Finally, the cohesion of the night shift team is also nurtured by moments shared outside the emergency department. Taking the time to get together to chat, exchange anecdotes or simply share a meal at the end of the shift strengthens the bonds between team members. These informal moments are just as important as professional interactions, as they enable you to get to know your colleagues better, build trust and develop a sense of camaraderie. They help to create a calmer working atmosphere and strengthen team spirit.

- **The psychological and emotional challenges of the night shift**
  ◦ **The loneliness and isolation of the night**

The loneliness and isolation of the night are omnipresent realities for orderlies and other healthcare professionals who work during these quiet, often silent hours. When day gives way to darkness, the rhythm of the hospital changes: the once bustling corridors empty out, the lights dim, and the sounds of daily activity become distant murmurs. In this setting, isolation and solitude can become constant companions, providing both unique challenges and moments of deep reflection.

One of the first aspects of nocturnal loneliness is the absence of the immediate support found during the day. Reduced staffing levels at night mean that exchanges with colleagues are less frequent, and responsibilities can weigh more heavily on individual team members. For the caregiver, this can translate into a feeling of isolation, especially when faced with complex or emotionally challenging situations without easy access to a doctor or other specialist colleagues. This professional solitude demands a high degree of autonomy and confidence in one's own skills, but it can also accentuate stress and anxiety, particularly when decisions have to be made quickly.

Night-time isolation can also have an impact on caregivers' emotional well-being. Working while the majority of the population is asleep can create a disconnect with the outside world, reinforcing the feeling of being "out of time" or on the margins of normal social life. This disconnect can be exacerbated by the lack of contact with family and friends, who live according to a diurnal rhythm. Emotional isolation can gradually set in, making it more difficult to maintain a balance between professional and personal life. For some, this sense of disconnection can lead to inner loneliness, a deeper form of isolation where we feel cut off not only from the outside world, but also from ourselves.

However, the loneliness of the night is not only negative. It can offer precious moments of calm and reflection, when caregivers can reconnect with their commitment and the raison d'être of their work. In the quiet of the night, it's possible to develop a more intimate relationship with patients, offering more attentive listening and more personalized support, away from the hustle and bustle of the day. These moments of solitude can become opportunities for more human-centred work, where every interaction takes on a deeper meaning.

What's more, nocturnal solitude can also be a time for introspection and personal growth. Isolation allows you to take stock of your journey, reflect on your motivations and step back from the challenges you face on a daily basis. It's a time to build resilience, refocus on what really matters, and develop personal stress management strategies. For some, these moments of solitude can even become a source of inner strength, providing the energy needed to keep moving forward in a sometimes difficult environment.

To cope with the loneliness and isolation of the night, it's essential to develop coping strategies. Maintaining regular contact with colleagues, even beyond working hours, can help reduce feelings of isolation. Taking part in support groups or social activities adapted to shift work can also help create a network of solidarity and sharing. The importance of emotional support should not be underestimated: talking about one's experiences with peers who understand the specific challenges of night work can bring relief and reassurance.

It's also crucial to look after your mental and physical health by establishing a routine that encourages rest, relaxation and reconnection with yourself. Practicing relaxation techniques, such as meditation or deep breathing, can help manage moments of intense loneliness. Similarly, taking the time to recharge your batteries, whether through reading, writing or creative hobbies, can offer a welcome escape and reinforce your sense of well-being.

○   **Managing emotional fatigue and burn-out**

Dealing with emotional fatigue and burn-out has become a key concern for healthcare professionals, especially those working night shifts. The demanding and often stressful nature of night work, combined with the specific challenges of caring for patients in an often silent and isolated environment, can quickly lead to deep emotional wear and tear. Emotional fatigue manifests itself as mental and emotional exhaustion, while burn-out represents a

97

more advanced state of psychological distress, characterized by a loss of motivation, a feeling of detachment, and a decline in work efficiency. To preserve their well-being and continue to provide quality care, caregivers must learn to recognize the warning signs of these conditions, and adopt strategies to prevent and manage them.

One of the first signs of emotional fatigue is a feeling of exhaustion that persists despite physical rest. This type of fatigue doesn't simply disappear with a good night's sleep or a day off; it's a deeper exhaustion, affecting the ability to concentrate, feel empathy, and cope with the daily challenges of the job. Caregivers may begin to feel disconnected from their patients, as if becoming insensitive to their suffering, or experience increased irritability towards colleagues or patients. These feelings are often accompanied by a sense of cynicism or frustration, where tasks that were once performed with care and commitment become meaningless routine obligations.

To prevent emotional fatigue and burn-out, it's crucial to develop an awareness of oneself and one's limits. Recognizing that you're overworked or starting to feel emotionally drained is the first step to taking corrective action. This may involve taking a break, delegating certain tasks, or asking colleagues or management for help. It's important to remember that asking for help is not a sign of weakness, but a proactive step towards preserving your mental health and continuing to work effectively.

Another essential strategy for managing emotional fatigue is to set up decompression routines. After a particularly strenuous night shift, it's helpful to take a moment to relax and refocus before heading home. This can include relaxation techniques such as deep breathing, meditation, or stretching, which help to release tension built up during the shift. It can also be beneficial to develop personal rituals for transitioning between work and home, such as listening to soothing music on the way or writing in a journal to express feelings and thoughts.

Work-life balance plays a crucial role in preventing burn-out. Working nights can upset this balance, but it's essential to find time for yourself, for your loved ones, and for activities that bring pleasure and rejuvenation. Cultivating hobbies, spending time with family and friends, or simply allowing yourself moments of solitude to rest and relax are effective ways of counterbalancing the stress of work. Maintaining an active social life, even outside normal working hours, helps reduce the sense of isolation often associated with night shifts, and reinforces the emotional support needed to cope with professional challenges.

It is also important to address emotional fatigue and burn-out within the care team. Encouraging a working environment where team members feel comfortable talking about their difficulties and sharing experiences is crucial. Regular debriefings, not only after critical situations, but also to discuss day-to-day issues, can provide a space for expressing concerns, sharing advice, and finding collective solutions to problems encountered. Solidarity between colleagues is an essential bulwark against burnout, as it allows us to feel understood and supported in difficult times.

Finally, if emotional fatigue or burn-out becomes too much to bear, it's essential not to hesitate to seek professional support. Consulting a psychologist, mental health counselor or coach can provide additional tools for managing stress, developing resilience strategies and regaining emotional balance. Professional support helps you take a step back, understand the root causes of burn-out, and implement lasting changes in the way you manage stress and responsibilities.

- **Maintaining a personal/professional life balance**
  - ◦ **The impact of night work on social and family life**

Night work has a significant impact on the social and family life of healthcare professionals, profoundly altering their rhythm of life and the way they connect with their loved ones. While necessary to ensure continuity of patient care, this staggered lifestyle can bring considerable personal and relational challenges. The consequences of these atypical schedules manifest themselves in various aspects of daily life, affecting social interactions, participation in family activities, and even the emotional health of caregivers.

One of the first effects of night work on social life is the gap with the rest of society. Working while most people are asleep, and sleeping while the world is awake, creates a kind of temporal gap between night carers and their friends, family and wider community. Opportunities to participate in social activities, such as dinners with friends, outings, or community events, become limited, as these activities often take place during the hours when caregivers are resting or preparing for their shift. This gap can lead to a feeling of isolation, where you feel on the bangs of the events that punctuate the lives of others.

From a family point of view, night work imposes specific constraints. Caregivers who work nights may find it difficult to be present for key moments in family life, such as family meals, children's homework, or weekend activities. This absence can be felt by both the caregiver and family members, creating an unintended emotional distance. For parents, the difficulty lies in having to juggle the needs of the family with the demands of night work, sometimes sacrificing their own rest to be available during the day. This situation can generate feelings of guilt, frustration and accumulated fatigue, making the management of family life more complex.

Night work can also affect a couple's relationship. The lack of synchronized schedules can reduce the amount of time spent together, making it difficult to maintain fluid, regular communication. Moments of sharing, which are essential to the solidity of a relationship, can become rarer, leading to a gradual erosion of complicity and emotional closeness. Couples often have to find strategies to maintain their bond, by planning specific times to spend together, or using communication technologies to stay connected despite shifting schedules.

In addition, night work can have an impact on the physical and mental health of caregivers, which in turn influences their social and family life. Sleep deprivation, disrupted circadian rhythms and accumulated exhaustion can lead to health problems such as chronic fatigue, reduced immunity and mood disorders. These effects can reduce caregivers' ability to participate actively in social and family life, further exacerbating feelings of isolation and disconnection. The stress associated with these constraints can also affect patience, tolerance and the ability to manage conflict, both at work and at home.

However, it is possible to find a balance, even when working nights. The key is to implement appropriate strategies to preserve social and family life. It's important to communicate openly with loved ones about the specific challenges and needs of working nights. This can include planning dedicated times for family and friends on days off, or creating rituals that keep you connected despite the shifting hours. For example, a parent working nights can establish a morning routine with their children before bedtime, or a couple can devote time to a joint activity on days off.

What's more, it's essential to take care of your physical and mental health so you can be fully present in your social and family life. This means keeping to a regular sleep schedule, adopting a balanced diet, and engaging in relaxing activities to manage stress. Finding support, whether through discussion groups with other night carers or through professional consultations, can also help to better manage the challenges associated with this lifestyle.

   ◦   **Strategies for a sustainable balance**
Strategies for sustainable balance are essential for caregivers, especially those who work night shifts, in order to reconcile their

professional and personal lives while preserving their mental and physical health. Working nights presents unique challenges that can disrupt normal life rhythms, affect sleep quality, and impact social and family relationships. To avoid burnout and maintain a harmonious balance, it's crucial to adopt strategies that effectively manage the demands of night work while cultivating lasting personal well-being.

One of the first strategies is to establish a rigorous and adapted sleep routine. Sleep is the pillar on which overall health rests, and for night workers it's vital to recreate an environment conducive to rest, even in broad daylight. This can include setting up a dark, quiet bedroom, using blackout curtains or a sleep mask to block out light, as well as earplugs or white noise to mask outside noises. It's also important to maintain a regular sleep schedule, even on days off, to stabilize the circadian rhythm and minimize fatigue. A short nap before starting the night shift can also help boost alertness and energy.

Another key strategy is to adopt a balanced, structured diet. Working nights can disrupt eating habits, and it's tempting to turn to quick snacks or sugar-rich foods to compensate for fatigue. However, a healthy, planned diet is crucial to maintaining energy and concentration. It's advisable to eat light, nutritious meals before the start of the shift, and to focus on healthy snacks during the night, such as fruit, nuts or vegetables. Avoiding caffeine at the end of the shift is also important to avoid disrupting post-shift sleep. Hydration is just as essential: drinking water regularly helps maintain alertness and prevent dehydration.

For a lasting balance, it's also essential to plan moments of disconnection and relaxation. The stress and pressure of night work can build up, and it's important to create spaces during the day to relax and recharge. Whether it's through regular physical activity, such as yoga or walking, which helps reduce stress and improve sleep quality, or through creative and soothing hobbies, it's crucial to set aside time for yourself. These moments of relaxation help to decompress after a demanding shift and maintain good mental health.

Maintaining active social ties is another vital component of lasting balance. Working nights can isolate caregivers from their usual social circle, and it's important to find ways to stay connected with family and friends. This can include planning activities on days off, making regular phone calls, or organizing social gatherings adapted to staggered schedules. These interactions reinforce emotional support and help maintain a sense of belonging, reducing feelings of isolation.

Organization and time management are also essential strategies for effectively balancing the different demands of life. It can be helpful to plan household chores, medical appointments and social activities in advance, taking into account necessary rest periods. Prioritizing tasks and delegating them where possible helps to reduce mental workload and focus on the most important aspects of life, both at work and at home.

Open communication with loved ones and the work team is another crucial strategy. Sharing the challenges of night work with the family, discussing specific needs and adjusting expectations create an environment of mutual understanding and support. Within the care team, fluid communication and mutual support strengthen cohesion and facilitate the management of stressful situations, thus contributing to a more balanced working environment.

Finally, it's essential to recognize your own limits and know when to ask for help. Working nights can be exhausting, and it's important to know when it's time to take a break, consult a health professional for advice on stress management, or join a support group to exchange ideas with others experiencing the same challenges. Preventing burn-out means paying constant attention to one's own well-being and using the resources available to maintain this balance.

Chapter 6

Career development and prospects

- **Career opportunities as an orderly**
  - **Becoming a night referent**

Becoming a night referent is a role of particular importance within care teams, especially in an environment as delicate and demanding as that of night work. Often perceived as a pillar of the team, the night referent is responsible for coordinating activities, supporting colleagues and ensuring continuity of care in a setting where resources may be limited and emergency situations more complex to manage. This role requires not only solid clinical expertise, but also leadership and communication skills, and the ability to handle stress and the unexpected calmly and effectively.

Assuming the role of night referral starts with recognition of the importance of the role. Unlike the daytime, when medical teams are more numerous and resources more readily available, the night is often marked by greater autonomy. The night referent thus becomes the reference person, the one to whom people turn for advice, to make quick decisions in emergency situations, or to solve problems that may arise in the absence of other managers. This responsibility demands great self-confidence, in-depth knowledge of care protocols, and the ability to make informed decisions even under pressure.

One of the first qualities needed to become a good night referral is a mastery of technical and clinical skills. This includes a thorough knowledge of common pathologies, emergency procedures, and the specific care of nocturnal patients. The referent must be able to supervise the care provided, quickly detect signs of deterioration in patients, and guide other team members in the application of medical protocols. This technical expertise is fundamental to inspiring the confidence of colleagues, and to ensuring that the care delivered during the night is of the same high quality as that delivered during the day.

In addition to technical skills, the role of Night Manager requires leadership skills. The referent must be able to motivate his or her team, maintain a positive working atmosphere and foster cohesion

106

within the group. This involves active listening, the ability to delegate tasks fairly, and ensuring that every team member feels supported and valued. Leadership at night is often more subtle than during the day: it relies on influence, persuasion and the ability to remain calm and reassuring, even in moments of tension.

Communication is another essential aspect of the night shift manager's role. The referent must ensure clear transmission of information between the different teams, particularly when handing over instructions between day and night shifts. He or she is also responsible for communication with doctors on call and emergency services, ensuring that crucial information on patients' condition is passed on accurately and efficiently. Good communication helps to avoid errors, coordinate interventions and ensure that all team members are on the same wavelength.

The night referent must also be flexible and adaptable. Hospital nights can be unpredictable, with rapidly changing situations requiring constant adjustments. The referent must be able to prioritize tasks, reorganize care according to emergencies, and remain vigilant in the face of the unexpected. This flexibility goes hand in hand with an ability to manage stress: as a leader, the referent must be a model of resilience, capable of maintaining composure and making informed decisions, even at the most critical moments.

Becoming a night shift supervisor also implies a commitment to continuous professional development. The referent must keep abreast of the latest developments in care, new medical technologies, and best practices in team management. They must also be willing to share their knowledge with colleagues, train newcomers, and encourage learning within the team. This commitment to training and continuous improvement is essential to ensure that the night shift functions optimally, and that patients receive the best possible care.

Last but not least, the role of night manager has an important emotional dimension. Working the night shift can be stressful, and it's essential that the referent is attuned to the emotional needs of his or her team. This can include offering moral support, helping to resolve conflicts, or simply being there for colleagues when they need it. A good referent knows that the quality of care also depends on the well-being of the team, and strives to create a working environment where everyone feels respected, supported and able to give their best.

○ **Further training**

Further training is essential for all healthcare professionals, and is particularly important for caregivers, especially those who work night shifts. In a constantly evolving field, where medical practices, technologies and care protocols are regularly renewed, ongoing training is essential to maintain a high level of competence, adapt to new requirements and offer quality care to patients. Beyond the acquisition of new skills, this approach reflects a commitment to professional excellence and personal development.

The pursuit of further training enables us to keep up to date with the latest advances in the medical and nursing fields. The health sciences are evolving rapidly, with the emergence of new therapies, innovative techniques and research that are changing care practices. Regular training ensures that caregivers and night nurses are not left behind by these developments, which is crucial if they are to apply care based on the best available evidence. For example, training in new resuscitation techniques, palliative care patient management or the latest infection control recommendations ensures that patients benefit from the safest, most effective interventions.

Further training also offers the opportunity to develop specialized skills. Depending on personal interests and the specific needs of the department, a caregiver may choose to specialize in a particular field, such as pain management, psychiatric care, or the care of the elderly. This specialization not only enriches the professional career, but also strengthens the caregiver's ability to intervene expertly in complex situations, bringing added value to the team and to patients. For example, training in palliative care provides invaluable skills for accompanying patients at the end of life, offering both technical and emotional support at particularly delicate moments.

Further training is also a way of preparing for new responsibilities or career development. For those aspiring to supervisory, coordination or management positions, training in management, communication or leadership is essential. They enable you to develop the skills needed to manage a team, handle crisis situations and communicate effectively with the various players in the healthcare sector. These skills are particularly important for night nurses, who often have to make autonomous decisions and manage small teams in a sometimes stressful environment. Training in these areas prepares caregivers to take on leadership roles, such as night referral, with confidence and competence.

Ongoing training also plays a crucial role in preventing burnout. Learning new things, feeling intellectually stimulated and seeing one's work evolve thanks to the skills acquired are all factors that help maintain motivation and commitment. Through training, caregivers can rediscover aspects of their profession that give them satisfaction and pride, which is essential if they are to remain fulfilled in a demanding career. In addition, training in stress management, resilience or relaxation techniques can provide invaluable tools to better manage the emotional and physical challenges of night work.

Further training is not just an individual initiative, but also contributes to the dynamism and overall quality of care within the team. A caregiver trained in new practices can share his or her knowledge with colleagues, enriching collective knowledge and improving the practices of the team as a whole. This dissemination of knowledge strengthens cohesion within the group, encourages mutual learning and ensures that all team members benefit from the latest advances in care.

Finally, the pursuit of further training is an expression of commitment to patients. By pursuing further training, caregivers show that they take to heart their responsibility to provide the best possible care, by keeping abreast of developments in their profession and constantly seeking to improve their skills. This commitment is recognized and appreciated by patients, who feel the difference in the quality of care they receive. For caregivers, knowing that they are doing everything in their power to be as competent and prepared as possible boosts job satisfaction and a sense of accomplishment.

- **Recognition and enhancement of the profession**
  - **The challenges of valuing night work**

The issues involved in valuing night work are manifold, and are of crucial importance to healthcare professionals who work this often overlooked and underestimated time slot. Working at night imposes particular challenges that go far beyond simple time constraints: it involves managing emergency situations with reduced resources, maintaining a high level of vigilance despite fatigue, and ensuring continuity of care in an environment where immediate support from colleagues and departments may be limited. Yet, despite these challenges, night shift work is often less valued than day shift work, both institutionally and in terms of social recognition. Valuing this work is therefore essential not only to improve working conditions for caregivers, but also to ensure optimum quality of care for patients.

One of the first challenges in valuing night work is to recognize the importance and complexity of this role. Night carers are often perceived as working "behind the scenes", but their contribution is essential to the smooth running of the hospital. They look after patients during their most vulnerable hours, ensure continuity of

110

treatment, and intervene rapidly in emergencies. Their role requires particular expertise, as they often have to make decisions independently, without the immediate support of a full medical team. Recognizing and valuing this expertise underlines the importance of night work, and reinforces its legitimacy.

The value of night work also requires better financial recognition. Working at night entails significant personal and social sacrifices, such as adapting to a staggered lifestyle, isolation from family and friends, and exposure to increased health risks. These constraints should be compensated by adequate remuneration, which reflects not only the difficulties inherent in night work, but also the competence and commitment of caregivers who choose or accept to work these hours. Appropriate financial recognition is a concrete sign that their work is valued, and can help reduce turnover in these often hard-to-fill positions.

Another issue in valuing night work is taking into account the health and well-being of caregivers. Working nights has well-documented physiological and psychological impacts, including sleep disturbances, mood disorders, and an increased risk of chronic illness. Valuing night work also means putting measures in place to protect caregivers' health. This can include regular medical monitoring programs, training in stress and sleep management, and scheduling arrangements that reduce the negative effects of night work, such as adapted rotation cycles or sufficient rest periods between shifts.

Night shift work also requires institutional and social recognition. It is important for night carers to be visible and valued within their establishments, for their work to be recognized at team meetings, and for them to be included in decision-making processes. All too often, important decisions are taken during the day, without taking into account the realities of night work. Giving night carers a voice, involving them in discussions about the organization of care, and ensuring that their specific needs and challenges are taken into account, are all part of institutional valuing.

Moreover, valuing night work has a direct impact on the quality of patient care. When night carers feel recognized and supported, they are more motivated, more committed, and more likely to deliver high-quality care. Conversely, a lack of recognition can lead to demotivation, burnout, and reduced quality of care. Valuing night work therefore also means investing in the safety and well-being of patients, by ensuring that they receive care of equal quality, whatever the time of day.

Finally, enhancing the value of night work helps to make these positions more attractive. Many caregivers are reluctant to work at night because of the difficulties involved, but appropriate recognition can make these positions more attractive. By offering specific benefits, such as ongoing training opportunities, night bonuses or flexible working hours, healthcare establishments can attract and retain competent, motivated professionals for these essential positions. Greater attractiveness translates into a more stable and experienced night shift team, which benefits the entire facility.

◦ How to claim your rights and improve your working conditions

Claiming one's rights and improving working conditions is a crucial issue for healthcare professionals, especially those working in demanding environments such as night shifts. Working in optimal conditions is essential not only for the quality of care provided to patients, but also for the well-being and satisfaction of caregivers themselves. To claim your rights and improve your working conditions effectively, it's important to follow a structured approach, combining communication, collective mobilization and the use of appropriate tools and bodies.

The first step in asserting your rights is to be familiar with them. It's essential to familiarize yourself with labor laws, collective bargaining agreements and agreements specific to your establishment. These documents define workers' rights, such as working hours, breaks, compensation for night work, vacations and safety conditions. A good knowledge of these rights enables you to better identify situations where they are not respected, and to formulate claims based on solid, legitimate arguments.

Once rights are known, it's important to observe and document problem situations. This may include inadequate working conditions, understaffing, excessive working hours, or breaches of safety regulations. Keeping a log of incidents, collecting evidence, and gathering testimonials from colleagues can be useful steps in supporting a claim. These concrete elements are invaluable for backing up a claim and demonstrating that current conditions do not meet expected standards.

Communication is an essential key to the grievance process. It's important to start by expressing your concerns clearly and constructively to your superiors. Asking for a meeting with your superior to discuss the problems encountered and propose solutions can be a first step. During this exchange, it is crucial to adopt a respectful but assertive tone, emphasizing the impact of working conditions on the quality of care and the well-being of caregivers. It can be useful to prepare for this discussion in advance, by listing the points to be addressed and the improvements desired.

If individual action isn't enough, collective mobilization becomes an essential strategy. Getting together with colleagues to discuss common problems and possible solutions helps to strengthen the weight of demands. Collective action is often more influential than individual action, because it shows that concerns are shared by a large number of people. Team meetings, general assemblies or informal discussion groups are effective ways of exchanging ideas, organizing collective action and deciding on next steps.

When it comes to collective mobilization, it's important to rely on unions or employee representatives. Their mission is to defend workers' rights, and they have the experience and tools needed to make demands. They can help formulate demands, organize actions, and negotiate with the employer. Calling on a trade union can provide legal and strategic support, and give greater weight to demands. Unions can also organize mediation or strikes if necessary, to make caregivers' voices heard.

Negotiation is a crucial stage in achieving concrete improvements in working conditions. In discussions with the employer or management, it is essential to adopt a constructive approach and propose realistic solutions. Rather than simply denouncing problems, it is useful to suggest alternatives, such as adjusting working hours, hiring additional staff, or improving safety conditions. Negotiations must aim for a compromise that respects caregivers' rights while taking into account the facility's constraints. The ability to negotiate effectively depends on rigorous preparation, clear communication and a willingness to find common ground.

If negotiations fail, other means of action may be considered. Petitions, open letters or awareness-raising campaigns are tools that can be used to alert public opinion or the relevant authorities to unacceptable working conditions. These actions can put additional pressure on the employer and encourage more open dialogue. However, it is important to conduct such actions within the law, and to maintain a constructive dialogue with the employer.

Finally, it is essential to remain committed to a process of continuous improvement of working conditions. Claiming one's rights is not a one-off action, but an ongoing process that needs to be adapted to changing working conditions. By getting actively involved in discussions on working conditions, keeping abreast of legislative developments, and participating in collective initiatives, caregivers can help create a fairer, safer and more fulfilling working environment.

- **The future of night work in hospitals**
  - ◦ **New technologies for night-time care**

New technologies are playing an increasingly central role in improving night-time care, offering tools and solutions that facilitate the work of caregivers and enhance the quality of patient care. Working at night presents specific challenges, such as the need to maintain constant vigilance despite fatigue, to manage emergency situations with limited resources, and to ensure continuity of care in an often quieter but potentially more unpredictable environment. Technological advances are providing effective responses to these challenges, by improving communication, optimizing patient monitoring, and increasing the efficiency of interventions.

One of the main contributions of new technologies to night care is improved patient monitoring. Modern monitoring systems enable real-time tracking of patients' vital signs, such as heart rate, oxygen saturation, blood pressure and respiration. These systems are often equipped with automatic alerts that signal any abnormal variations, enabling caregivers to intervene quickly, even in the event of subtle changes. This continuous monitoring is particularly valuable at night, when patients are asleep and signs of deterioration may go unnoticed without extra vigilance. In this way, new technologies help reduce the risk of adverse events and ensure that critical situations are dealt with rapidly.

Communication technologies have also transformed night work, facilitating exchanges between care team members and emergency services. Internal communication systems, such as digital pagers, secure smartphones and instant messaging platforms, enable caregivers to stay connected at all times, exchange information in real time, and coordinate interventions efficiently. In the event of an emergency, these tools make it possible to rapidly mobilize the necessary resources, inform on-call doctors or response teams, and ensure that all team members are on the same wavelength. Fluid communication is essential for effective night care management, and new technologies offer solutions that make this communication faster, more accurate, and more secure.

Wearable, connected medical devices are another technological innovation enhancing night-time care. Patients can be equipped with wearable sensors that monitor various health parameters, such as blood glucose for diabetics or oxygen saturation for patients with respiratory disorders. These devices send real-time data to caregivers, enabling them to monitor patients' health status without having to disturb them. For caregivers, this means fewer interruptions to patients' sleep, more discreet monitoring, and the ability to anticipate needs before they become urgent. These technologies enhance patient autonomy while providing continuous monitoring, even in a nocturnal care setting.

Electronic medical records (EMRs) are also a major asset for night care. These systems centralize all a patient's medical information, enabling caregivers to quickly and easily access crucial data such as medical history, allergies, prescriptions and test results. At night, when staff numbers are low and access to medical specialists may be limited, EMRs enable informed decisions to be made based on complete, up-to-date information. Caregivers can also document care given, vital signs taken and clinical observations in real time, ensuring continuity and traceability of care.

Robotic innovations are also beginning to find their way into night-time care. Assistance robots, for example, can be used to carry out certain repetitive tasks, such as dispensing medication, transporting medical equipment or accompanying patients over short distances. These robots free up time for caregivers, enabling them to concentrate on the more complex, human aspects of their work. In addition, robots can be used to monitor corridors and rooms, detecting any unusual movement or behavior, such as a patient falling or needing assistance. This automated surveillance adds an extra layer of security, particularly useful during hours when staff numbers are low.

Finally, online training and simulation platforms offer caregivers the possibility of continuous training, even when working at night. These tools provide access to interactive training modules, simulations of emergency situations, and educational resources tailored to the specific needs of night-time work. Ongoing training is essential to maintain a high level of competence, and these technologies enable caregivers to perfect their skills at their own pace, taking into account their staggered working hours. What's more, realistic simulators offer a valuable opportunity to practice complex procedures or crisis management, boosting the confidence and preparedness of night shifts.

○ **Legislative and organizational developments**

Legislative and organizational changes play a central role in the continuous improvement of the healthcare system, particularly for professionals working in demanding environments such as night services. These changes, driven by the need to ensure quality of care, patient safety and the well-being of caregivers, are gradually transforming professional practices, working conditions and the organization of care. Understanding and adapting to these changes is essential for caregivers, not only to meet regulatory requirements, but also to play an active part in improving the healthcare system as a whole.

On the legislative front, several reforms have been introduced to provide a better framework for night work and protect caregivers. In particular, these reforms aim to ensure that working conditions for night carers are commensurate with the specific challenges they face. For example, working time legislation imposes precise limits on the length of night shifts, emphasizing the importance of adequate rest periods to prevent exhaustion and burn-out. These regulations also include provisions on breaks and financial compensation, such as wage supplements for night work, which recognize the personal sacrifices and additional demands associated with these schedules. These legislative measures help to create a safer and fairer working environment for carers, ensuring that their rights are respected and their well-being taken into account.

At the same time, legislative changes have also been introduced to reinforce patient safety and ensure that the quality of care remains high, whatever the time of day or night. Legislation governing the ongoing training of caregivers, for example, aims to ensure that the skills of healthcare professionals are constantly updated. This is particularly important for night staff, who often have to make autonomous decisions and manage emergency situations with limited resources. In addition, regulations require healthcare facilities to maintain sufficient staffing levels to meet patients' needs efficiently and safely, even during the night. These measures are designed to minimize the risk of medical error and guarantee continuous quality care.

On the organizational front, recent developments have focused on optimizing care coordination and human resources management. The organization of teamwork has been rethought to better respond to the specificities of night-time work. For example, the introduction of pairs of nursing assistants and nurses strengthens cooperation and ensures that care is delivered in an efficient and consistent manner. In addition, roles and responsibilities are often redefined to ensure that each member of the night shift team knows precisely what his or her tasks are, and can carry them out in the best possible conditions.

The integration of new technologies is also a key aspect of organizational developments. Digital tools, such as electronic medical records and internal communication systems, have been widely adopted to facilitate night care management. These technologies make it possible not only to centralize and share information in real time, but also to coordinate interventions more fluidly and efficiently. For example, automated alert systems can provide immediate warning of any deterioration in a patient's condition, enabling rapid intervention and reducing the risks associated with working at night.

Organizational developments are also aimed at improving the well-being of caregivers by taking into account their specific needs. Psychological support programs, stress management training and initiatives to improve the working environment are increasingly integrated into the policies of healthcare establishments. These initiatives aim to prevent burnout, promote a better work-life balance, and create a more humane working environment that is more respectful of caregivers' needs.

Finally, it is important to note that these legislative and organizational changes are often the fruit of consultation between the various players in the healthcare system: regulatory authorities, healthcare professionals, unions and care facilities. This collaboration ensures that the reforms implemented are both realistic and adapted to local needs. It also ensures that caregivers have a voice in the decisions that affect their day-to-day work, which is essential to ensure the buy-in and commitment of teams in implementing these changes.

120

Chapter 7
Risk and Safety Management on Night Shifts

- **Risks specific to night work**
  - **The risks of isolation and downsizing**

The risks associated with isolation and downsizing are crucial issues in healthcare, particularly for professionals working night shifts. These two factors, often interconnected, can have serious consequences not only for the quality of care delivered to patients, but also for the well-being of caregivers themselves. Isolation, when combined with downsizing, exacerbates the daily challenges faced by caregivers, increasing the risk of errors, overwork and burnout.

Isolation is a major problem for caregivers, especially those who work at night. Due to the reduced number of staff during these hours, caregivers can find themselves dealing with complex situations without the immediate support of colleagues or superiors. This isolation can make decision-making more difficult, as the caregiver often has to act alone, without the opportunity to consult or delegate. Professional solitude also increases stress and anxiety, as the sense of responsibility becomes greater when you're the only one looking after patients' safety. This isolation can also lead to a feeling of discouragement or disengagement, especially if caregivers feel that their night work is not properly recognized by the day team or hierarchy.

Downsizing, often motivated by budgetary constraints, further exacerbates these risks. With fewer staff available, each caregiver is entrusted with a greater number of tasks and responsibilities. The workload becomes heavier, increasing fatigue and the risk of errors. In emergency situations, this downsizing can have dramatic consequences: response to critical situations may be delayed, basic care may be neglected, and patients may be left without the necessary supervision. Downsizing also limits the scope for individualized care, as caregivers have to concentrate on the most urgent tasks, often to the detriment of listening to and accompanying patients.

The consequences of isolation and downsizing are not limited to the immediate impact on the care provided; they also affect the mental and physical health of caregivers. Overwork can lead to burnout, characterized by intense fatigue, growing cynicism and reduced work efficiency. This burn-out can manifest itself in physical symptoms such as sleep disorders, headaches or muscle pain, as well as emotional symptoms such as irritability, sadness or feelings of incompetence. If nothing is done to remedy these conditions, caregivers may end up leaving their posts, further exacerbating downsizing and creating a vicious circle.

Isolation and downsizing can also undermine the cohesion of the care team. When staff numbers are reduced, communication between team members becomes more difficult, as everyone is focused on their own tasks and has less time to exchange ideas with colleagues. This can lead to team fragmentation, with caregivers feeling isolated not only physically, but socially too. The loss of cohesion and mutual support between colleagues can reduce motivation and make work even harder. What's more, a lack of communication and coordination can increase the risk of errors, as crucial patient information may not be properly shared.

To address these risks, it is essential that healthcare facilities take steps to support their caregivers and ensure patient safety. This can include adjusting staffing levels in line with actual needs, ensuring that caregivers are not overloaded and have the resources they need to do their jobs effectively. Technology can also play an important role, helping to compensate for certain repetitive tasks or facilitating communication between team members, even at a distance.

Strengthening psychological and emotional support for caregivers is also crucial. This can take the form of support programs, stress management training, or the creation of opportunities for sharing and debriefing among colleagues. Fostering a culture of solidarity and mutual support within the team can help mitigate the effects of isolation and strengthen resilience in the face of the challenges posed by downsizing.

○ **Risk of violence or aggression (patients, visitors)**
The risk of violence or aggression, whether from patients or visitors, is a major concern for healthcare professionals, especially those who work night shifts. The very nature of night work, often marked by fewer staff, less supervision, and a quieter but potentially more tense atmosphere, can increase caregivers' vulnerability to such behavior. Understanding these risks and putting strategies in place to prevent them is essential to ensuring the safety of caregivers and maintaining a calm, respectful working environment.

Aggression in healthcare facilities can take many forms, from verbal abuse to physical violence. Patients themselves can become aggressive, often as a result of their condition, pain, confusion or mental disorder. Patients suffering from dementia, psychiatric disorders or under the influence of substances can be particularly unpredictable, reacting violently to situations they perceive as stressful or threatening. At night, when there are fewer staff and the environment is calmer, these behaviors may go unnoticed until they reach a critical point, making crisis management more complex.

Visitors, whether family members or friends of patients, can also be a source of tension. They may be stressed or emotional because of their loved one's medical situation, and this stress can sometimes turn to aggression, especially if their expectations are not met or if they perceive slowness or incompetence in care. Frustration can quickly escalate into conflict, putting caregivers in a difficult position, especially at night, when procedures for calling in reinforcements may be less responsive.

Reduced staffing levels, common during night-time hours, exacerbate these risks. Fewer staff often means fewer witnesses or interveners to defuse tense situations before they escalate into violence. The lack of immediate support can also make caregivers more reluctant to intervene proactively when they sense a situation is deteriorating, for fear of not being able to manage the consequences alone. In addition, physical isolation in certain areas of the facility can make caregivers more vulnerable, with limited access to help in times of urgent need.

The consequences of violence or aggression are not only physical, although injury is obviously a direct risk. There are also significant psychological consequences for caregivers. Being a victim or witness of aggression can lead to post-traumatic stress, heightened anxiety and reduced job satisfaction. In the long term, these experiences can lead to burnout, emotional disengagement and even resignation, making the situation even worse by further downsizing and increasing the workload for those who remain.

To deal with these risks, it is essential that healthcare establishments put in place clear and effective violence prevention policies. This starts with training caregivers to manage aggressive behavior, teaching them to recognize warning signs, de-escalate tensions and use de-escalation techniques. Such training should include simulations and role-playing exercises, so that caregivers feel prepared to react appropriately when confronted with aggression.

Facilities must also ensure that safety protocols are in place and accessible to all caregivers, day and night. This includes means of emergency communication, such as portable panic buttons, radios or cell phones, so that help can be summoned quickly. In addition, the presence of security personnel, even if reduced, can have a deterrent effect on aggressive behavior and offer immediate support in the event of an incident. Particularly sensitive areas, such as emergency rooms or psychiatric wards, should be specially monitored, with video surveillance systems and strict access control.

At the same time, it is crucial to promote a culture of support within the healthcare team. Caregivers need to know that they can count on their colleagues and superiors to support them when things go wrong. This can involve regular meetings where incidents are discussed openly, without blame, to learn lessons and improve safety protocols. Psychological support after an attack is also fundamental, with access to counseling or therapy services to help caregivers overcome trauma and regain confidence in their ability to carry out their job safely.

- **Safety protocols to be implemented**
  - ◦ **Fire safety and night-time evacuation**

Fire safety and night-time evacuation are crucial aspects of risk management in healthcare facilities, where the safety of patients, carers and other staff must be ensured in all circumstances, including during the hours of darkness. At night, fire safety challenges are exacerbated by several factors: reduced staffing levels, patients often asleep or in vulnerable situations, reduced visibility, and reactivity potentially impaired by fatigue. These conditions make it all the more crucial to prepare, train and implement clear, effective protocols to ensure rapid, safe evacuation in the event of fire.

One of the first priorities in ensuring night-time fire safety is to install high-performance, regularly-maintained detection and alarm systems. Smoke, heat and gas detectors must be strategically placed in all critical areas of the facility, including patient rooms, corridors, treatment rooms and storage areas. These systems must be able to detect the slightest signs of fire and trigger an alarm powerful enough to wake caregivers and patients without delay. In addition, alarms must be linked to a centralized system that automatically notifies the emergency services, reducing response time in the event of a disaster.

Effective night-time evacuation relies heavily on staff preparation and training. Every member of the night shift must be fully trained in evacuation procedures, knowing exactly what role to play in the event of an emergency. This training must include regular drills, which simulate fire situations under realistic conditions. These drills are essential to train caregivers to act quickly and calmly, following predefined protocols. They also

126

help to identify and correct any shortcomings in evacuation plans, whether in terms of the layout of emergency exits, the allocation of responsibilities, or internal communication.

Communication is a key element in a night-time evacuation. In the event of a fire, it's vital that information flows quickly and clearly between all staff members, to effectively coordinate evacuation efforts. Caregivers need to be able to communicate not only with each other, but also with patients, to reassure them and guide them to the emergency exits. Emergency communication systems, such as walkie-talkies or intercoms, can be essential to maintain the link between different points in the facility, especially if certain areas become inaccessible due to smoke or flames.

Evacuating patients, especially those in vulnerable situations, is another major challenge during a night-time fire. Many patients may be unable to move about on their own due to their state of health, age or disability. It is therefore crucial that night staff are trained in the use of specific evacuation equipment, such as evacuation chairs, transfer sheets or stretchers. Each floor or department must have a sufficient supply of such equipment, and caregivers must know how to use it quickly and effectively. In addition, it is important to prioritize the evacuation of patients according to their state of health, ensuring that those most at risk are evacuated first.

Evacuation plans must be clearly posted in all parts of the establishment, indicating emergency exits, assembly points and routes to be followed in the event of an emergency. These plans must be clearly visible and understandable to all, including visitors who may be present at night. Emergency exits must be regularly checked to ensure that they are unobstructed and that doors open easily. Corridors and stairways must be well lit, even in the event of a power cut, thanks to efficient emergency lighting.

The management of fire containment systems is also crucial. Fire doors, fire-resistant partitions and smoke ventilation systems must be in place to limit the spread of flames and smoke, thus saving valuable evacuation time. Caregivers must be trained in the use of these devices, and know when and how to activate them to protect patients and staff.

Finally, after evacuation, it's important to organize the gathering and care of evacuated patients. Assembly points must be located at a sufficient distance from the building to guarantee the safety of evacuees. Staff must take a quick census to ensure that no one has been forgotten, and to organize medical care for any patients who need it. Once the fire has been brought under control, a debriefing is essential to analyze the response to the incident, identify areas for improvement, and adjust evacuation protocols if necessary.

- ○ **Managing high-risk situations (psychiatric patients, agitated patients)**

Managing high-risk situations, particularly with psychiatric or agitated patients, is an essential part of a carer's job, especially on night shifts where resources are often limited and the challenges magnified by loneliness and fatigue. Patients suffering from psychiatric disorders or confusion can, at any time, become unpredictable, displaying aggressive, agitated or dangerous behavior to themselves and others. Managing these situations effectively requires not only technical skills and a thorough knowledge of protocols, but also great empathy, the ability to remain calm, and a mastery of de-escalation techniques.

Patients with psychiatric disorders or in a state of extreme agitation may display a variety of risk behaviors, such as verbal or physical aggression, self-harm or even suicidal behavior. These behaviors can be triggered by a number of factors: an exacerbation of their illness, side effects of medication, confusion due to the hospital environment, or fear. At night, these situations can become even more complex to manage, due to the surrounding quiet, which can intensify the patient's sense of isolation and worsen their state of distress.

The first step in managing these situations is early identification of signs of deterioration or agitation. Caregivers must be particularly attentive to changes in behavior, signs of confusion, paranoia, motor agitation or incoherent speech. Spotting these signs early enables intervention before the situation becomes critical. A rapid assessment of the patient's condition, taking into account his or her medical history, current state and potential stressors, is essential to guide the most appropriate response.

Communication plays a key role in managing agitated or psychiatric patients. A calm, reassuring and non-threatening approach is crucial to defusing the situation. Caregivers should use simple, clear language, and avoid condescending or authoritarian attitudes. It's important to validate the patient's feelings, show that they are understood, and assure them that their well-being is the priority. Sometimes, simply speaking softly and reducing external stimuli, such as dimming the lights or moving other patients away, can help calm a patient in crisis.

The use of de-escalation techniques is also essential. These are strategies for reducing tension and preventing the escalation of violence. This can include managing the patient's personal space by maintaining a safe distance, adopting a non-threatening posture, and offering simple choices to give the patient a sense of control. For example, offering the patient a quiet place to sit or a glass of water can divert his or her attention from the immediate source of stress. Caregivers need to remain alert to any changes in the patient's behavior that might indicate escalating agitation, and be ready to adjust their approach accordingly.

In some cases, despite all efforts at de-escalation, it may be necessary to resort to more direct interventions to protect the patient and others. This may include the administration of sedative drugs, always under the supervision of a physician, or, as a last resort, the use of physical restraint measures. However, these interventions must be used with great caution and always as a last resort, respecting strict ethical and legal protocols. The aim is to minimize danger while respecting the patient's dignity and rights.

Collaboration with the multidisciplinary team is another crucial element in managing high-risk situations. Even if the night shift is often small, it is important to enlist the help of other healthcare professionals, such as psychiatric nurses, psychologists or doctors on call, whenever possible. Working as part of a team enables responsibilities to be shared, skills to be combined, and ensures that all management options are explored. Communication between team members must be constant and clear, particularly to ensure that everyone is kept informed of developments and decisions.

After the crisis has been managed, it is essential to assess and monitor the patient. Understanding the triggers of the crisis and the factors that contributed to the agitation helps prevent recurrences and adapt the patient's care plan. Psychological follow-up is often necessary to help patients manage their condition and prevent future crises. In addition, a debriefing with the team allows us to look back on the intervention, analyze what worked and what could be improved, and reinforce preparation for similar situations in the future.

Finally, it's important to recognize the emotional impact these situations can have on the caregivers themselves. Dealing with agitated or violent patients can be stressful and exhausting. Caregivers need to have access to psychological support and regular supervision to discuss difficult situations and receive advice on how to manage their own stress. The mental health of caregivers is essential if they are to continue providing quality care, even under difficult conditions.

- **The importance of ongoing risk management training**
  - **First aid and crisis management training**

Training in first aid and crisis management is essential for all healthcare professionals, but is particularly important for those working in hospitals, especially on night shifts. This training enables caregivers to react effectively and calmly to emergency situations, guaranteeing patient safety and continuity of care even at the most critical times. Mastering these skills is not limited to technical knowledge; it also involves developing the ability to manage stress, make rapid decisions and coordinate interventions under pressure.

First aid is the foundation of immediate care in a medical emergency. They include simple but vital actions such as cardiopulmonary resuscitation (CPR), airway clearance, stopping bleeding, and management of anaphylactic shock or cardiac arrest. When performed correctly and within the first few minutes of an incident, these actions can save lives. For caregivers, mastery of these techniques is essential, as they are often the first to intervene while waiting for a specialized medical team to arrive. The speed and effectiveness of these first actions can determine the outcome of a critical situation.

First aid training needs to be regularly updated to keep caregivers up to date with the latest recommendations and techniques. Periodic review of skills is essential to maintain a high level of preparedness, as protocols evolve with new medical knowledge. What's more, such training boosts caregivers' confidence in their ability to intervene, which is crucial when faced with unexpected situations. Emergency simulations, which reproduce realistic and stressful conditions, are particularly useful in preparing caregivers to act effectively under pressure. These exercises enable them to practice coordinating team interventions, communicating clearly and applying protocols smoothly and instinctively.

Crisis management goes beyond first aid. It encompasses the ability to rapidly assess an emergency situation, identify priorities, and orchestrate a coordinated response involving multiple stakeholders. Crises can arise unexpectedly and take many forms: a fire, an assault, a necessary evacuation, or a critical equipment failure. Each of these situations calls for a specific response, but all require rapid decision-making, effective communication, and optimal management of available resources.

Crisis management training focuses on team coordination, communication and decision-making under pressure. It includes learning clear and concise communication techniques, essential to avoid misunderstandings and ensure that each team member fully understands his or her role and responsibilities. Crisis management also involves familiarity with institutional protocols, such as evacuation plans, emergency call procedures, and the use of internal communication systems. Caregivers must be able to activate these protocols quickly and adapt them to the particular situation they are faced with.

Another crucial aspect of crisis management is stress management. Crises are, by definition, moments of high tension, when the ability to remain calm and focused is put to the test. Stress management training teaches caregivers techniques for maintaining composure, such as controlled breathing, focusing on the tasks at hand, and using mantras or positive thoughts to keep the situation under control. Learning to manage stress not only helps you to react better in the moment, but also prevents long-term emotional exhaustion, which can occur after particularly stressful interventions.

Crisis management doesn't end with resolving the immediate emergency. It also includes post-crisis debriefing, a process where teams look back on the event to analyze what went well, what could be improved, and to share their experiences and emotions. Debriefing is crucial for collective learning and for strengthening future preparedness. It helps to correct any shortcomings in protocols, to highlight the strengths of the response, and to support caregivers emotionally, offering them a space to express their feelings and receive the support they need.

Finally, training in crisis management and first-aid techniques strengthens the overall resilience of the care team. Knowing that they are well prepared to deal with critical situations, caregivers can approach their work with greater serenity and confidence. This preparation helps to create a working environment where patient safety is maximized, caregivers feel supported and competent, and the effectiveness of interventions is guaranteed, even in moments of greatest tension.

◦ The importance of regular simulations and exercises

The importance of regular simulations and exercises in the healthcare environment cannot be overstated, especially for professionals working in environments where emergency situations are frequent. These simulations and exercises are essential pedagogical tools that enable caregivers to train under conditions close to reality, perfect their technical skills, reinforce their ability to work as a team, and improve their responsiveness to the unexpected. They play a crucial role in preparing teams to effectively manage critical situations, thereby guaranteeing patient safety and quality of care.

Simulations provide a safe environment in which caregivers can practice techniques such as cardiopulmonary resuscitation (CPR), intubation and airway management, without the risks associated with real-life intervention. These exercises enable precise gestures to be rehearsed until they become automatic, which is vital in emergency situations where every second counts. For example, in a cardiac arrest simulation, caregivers can practice coordinating their actions, applying protocols smoothly, and using medical equipment with precision. This repeated practice improves not only individual skills, but also team cohesion, as everyone learns to work in synergy with their colleagues.

Regular drills are also essential to maintain a high level of vigilance and to ensure that caregivers stay up to date with the latest practices and protocols. Theoretical knowledge acquired during training courses can fade over time, especially if it is not regularly put into practice. Simulations help to refresh this knowledge, correct errors before they occur in a real-life context, and boost caregivers' confidence in their ability to intervene in any situation. For example, a crisis management simulation exercise, such as an emergency evacuation due to fire, ensures that every team member knows evacuation protocols, exit routes, and their precise role in the process.

The ability to manage stress is another fundamental aspect of simulations. By reproducing pressurized working conditions, these exercises enable caregivers to get used to dealing with the stress associated with emergency situations. When a real incident occurs, those who have regularly taken part in simulations are better prepared to remain calm, think clearly and make rapid decisions. Simulations create a space where caregivers can familiarize themselves with their own reactions to stress, learn how to manage them, and develop strategies to maintain their effectiveness, even in the most critical moments.

Simulations and regular exercises also play an important role in the continuous improvement of practices. Each simulation is a learning opportunity, not only for the direct participants, but also for the whole team. After each exercise, a debriefing is essential to analyze what went well, what could be improved, and to discuss weak points to be strengthened. These discussions enable valuable lessons to be learned, protocols to be adjusted, and solutions to be put in place to overcome any shortcomings identified. Debriefing also fosters a spirit of collaboration and open communication within the team, reinforcing cohesion and mutual trust.

In addition, simulations can be used to test and evaluate the effectiveness of protocols and equipment in a controlled environment. They offer a unique opportunity to identify potential weaknesses in existing systems, such as hardware failures, inconsistencies in procedures, or additional training needs. For example, a simulated power failure in a hospital may reveal shortcomings in emergency procedures, such as inadequate backup generators or a lack of staff training in blackout protocols. By identifying these problems during an exercise, healthcare facilities can take proactive steps to correct them before a real situation arises.

Regular simulations and exercises also have a positive impact on caregivers' morale and satisfaction. By offering them opportunities for ongoing training and skills enhancement, caregivers feel valued and supported by their organization. They gain greater confidence in their abilities, which translates into better job performance and greater job satisfaction. What's more, these exercises reinforce the feeling of belonging to a competent, well-prepared team, which is essential for maintaining good group dynamics and a positive working environment.

In conclusion, regular simulations and exercises are indispensable tools for preparing caregivers to deal with emergency situations competently, calmly and effectively. They help to perfect technical gestures, reinforce stress management, improve team coordination, and keep protocols up to date. By investing in these exercises, healthcare establishments ensure that their teams are ready to react optimally, guaranteeing patient safety and quality of care, even in the most critical situations. These practices also contribute to the professional satisfaction of caregivers, offering them the means to flourish in their role while ensuring their ongoing development.

136

Chapter 8

Psychological Impact and Long-Term Stress Management

- **The long-term psychological effects of night work**
  - **Sleep disorders and their impact on mental health**

Sleep disorders are a common reality for many healthcare professionals, particularly those who work night shifts or shift work. This imbalance in circadian rhythm, due to the inversion of sleep-wake cycles, can have profound consequences on mental health. Sleep plays a fundamental role in regulating our emotions, managing stress and maintaining our psychological well-being. When it is chronically disrupted, the repercussions can be significant, affecting not only quality of life, but also the ability to perform one's job effectively.

Sleep is essential for proper brain function. It is during phases of deep sleep that the brain consolidates memory, regenerates nerve cells, and eliminates metabolic waste accumulated during the day. When sleep is insufficient or of poor quality, these processes are compromised, which can lead to cognitive fatigue, reduced concentration and memory problems. For a caregiver, whose job demands constant attention, rapid decision-making and rigorous task management, these effects can significantly increase the risk of medical error, putting patient safety at risk.

Sleep disorders are also closely linked to mood and emotional health. Sleep deprivation can accentuate feelings of frustration, irritability and stress. It can make caregivers more sensitive to interpersonal tensions and daily work challenges, reducing their resilience in the face of stress. Over the long term, these disorders can lead to more severe mood disorders, such as anxiety or depression. The link between sleep and emotional regulation is well established: disturbed sleep can worsen symptoms of anxiety and depression, while these mood disorders can in turn make sleep even more difficult, creating a vicious circle that's hard to break.

Working nights or shifts can also disrupt social rhythms, increasing feelings of isolation and alienation. Caregivers may feel disconnected from family, friends and society in general, as their schedules do not coincide with those of others. This social disconnection can have a negative impact on mental health, exacerbating feelings of loneliness and emotional exhaustion. Lack of social support is a major risk factor for the development of psychological disorders, as it deprives individuals of the emotional resources needed to cope with stress.

Disturbed sleep also affects the body's physiology, which can indirectly affect mental health. For example, chronic sleep deprivation is associated with increased levels of the stress hormone cortisol, which can disrupt the overall hormonal balance and contribute to increased stress and anxiety. In addition, insufficient sleep is linked to appetite dysregulation, which can lead to weight gain, metabolic disorders and reduced physical energy. These physiological changes can worsen feelings of fatigue and general malaise, accentuating symptoms of depression and anxiety.

For caregivers, managing sleep disorders is therefore crucial to preserving their mental health and their ability to carry out their job competently and compassionately. It's important to put strategies in place to improve sleep quality, even when working shift work. This can include establishing regular sleep routines, even on days off, to stabilize circadian rhythm. Creating a sleep-friendly environment, using blackout curtains, earplugs and avoiding screens before bedtime, can also help improve sleep quality.

Adopting stress management techniques such as meditation, progressive muscle relaxation or yoga can also be beneficial. These practices help to calm the mind and body, making it easier to fall asleep and improving sleep quality. It may also be helpful to consult a healthcare professional for specific advice or treatment for sleep disorders, such as Cognitive Behavioural Therapy for Insomnia (CBT-I), which has been shown to be effective in treating chronic sleep disorders.

◦ **Effects on social and family life**

The effects of working shifts, particularly at night, on social and family life are profound and often underestimated. For caregivers working in environments where working hours are reversed compared to the majority of the population, reconciling professional and personal life can become a constant challenge. This time difference disrupts not only biological rhythms, but also social and family dynamics, creating a gap that is sometimes difficult to bridge between caregivers and their loved ones.

One of the first effects of night work on social life is the gradual disconnection from the social events and activities that punctuate most people's lives. Moments of conviviality, meetings with friends, family outings or even simple shared meals become difficult to organize when work schedules don't coincide with those of others. This repeated absence of socializing moments can lead to a feeling of isolation, where the caregiver feels on the margins of normal social life. This situation can lead to frustration and even sadness, due to the feeling of being "out of time", unable to participate in the social rituals that strengthen bonds with others.

On the family front, the repercussions can be just as significant. For parents, working nights often means missing out on important moments with their children, such as family meals, playtime or evening discussions. This absence, even if motivated by professional reasons, can be painfully felt by both parent and children. Children may feel a sense of lack or incomprehension, while parents may feel guilty or disconnected from their children's lives. Night shifts can also affect a couple's relationship, reducing moments of sharing and complicity. Staggered schedules can limit daily interactions, making communication and relationship maintenance more difficult. The lack of synchronized schedules can also create an emotional distance between partners, accentuating feelings of isolation.

Fatigue due to night work exacerbates these effects. Lack of sleep, combined with a disrupted circadian rhythm, can diminish a caregiver's energy and emotional availability. After a night's work, it is often difficult to find the energy to participate fully in family or social activities, even when schedules allow. This fatigue can lead to increased irritability, reduced patience and less commitment to social and family relationships. Caregivers may find themselves having to make difficult choices between resting to recuperate and spending time with loved ones, which can, in the long term, damage the quality of relationships.

To mitigate these effects, it is essential to implement strategies that help maintain a balance between professional and personal life. Open and honest communication with family and friends is an important first step. Explaining the constraints of night work, sharing your feelings and listening to those of others can help create mutual understanding and find appropriate solutions. For example, planning specific times to spend with family or friends, even if they don't fit in with traditional working hours, can help preserve bonds. Organizing quality activities, even short ones, can compensate in part for time lost due to work schedules.

It's also crucial to take care of your physical and mental health, so you can fully enjoy the time you spend with your loved ones. This can include establishing strict sleep routines, adopting a healthy diet and incorporating relaxing activities into the day. By maintaining a healthy energy level, caregivers can better cope with the demands of the night shift while remaining present for family and friends.

Finally, it can be helpful to seek support, whether through support groups for night workers, community activities adapted to staggered working hours, or by consulting a health professional to manage stress and fatigue. These resources can offer additional strategies for better reconciling work and personal life, and mitigating negative impacts on social and family life.

- **Stress management strategies for the night carer**
  - **Relaxation and stress management techniques**

Relaxation and stress management techniques have become indispensable in modern life, especially for healthcare professionals, who are often faced with high-pressure situations and an intense work rhythm. Stress, if not properly managed, can have devastating consequences on physical and mental health, leading to burnout, sleep disorders and a reduced quality of life. Adopting effective relaxation techniques not only helps to better manage daily stress, but also to restore inner balance, build resilience in the face of challenges and maintain optimal performance at work.

One of the most accessible and effective relaxation techniques is deep breathing. Deep breathing, or diaphragmatic breathing, involves breathing slowly and deeply, using the diaphragm rather than the chest. This reduces heart rate, lowers blood pressure and promotes a state of calm. When stress arises, taking a few minutes to concentrate on slow, controlled breathing can quickly soothe the body and mind. This technique is particularly useful in crisis situations, where the ability to remain calm and focused is essential.

Mindfulness meditation is another powerful method for managing stress. This practice involves focusing on the present moment, observing thoughts, emotions and sensations without judgment. Mindfulness meditation helps to develop a heightened awareness of oneself and one's environment, which can reduce automatic reactions to stress and increase the ability to handle difficult situations with greater serenity. Practicing mindfulness regularly, even for just a few minutes a day, can have significant effects on mental well-being, helping to reduce anxiety, improve concentration and strengthen emotional resilience.

Progressive muscle relaxation is another effective relaxation technique. It involves progressively contracting and then releasing different muscle groups in the body, starting with the feet and working up to the head. This practice helps to release accumulated physical tension and induce a state of deep relaxation. It is particularly beneficial for carers who spend long hours on their feet, or who experience work-related muscular pain. By practicing progressive muscle relaxation, we learn to better identify signs of tension in the body and release them before they become a source of stress or pain.

Yoga, which combines physical postures, breathing exercises and meditation, is another highly beneficial relaxation technique. Yoga helps to strengthen the body, improve flexibility and reduce physical tension, while calming the mind. By practicing yoga regularly, caregivers can develop greater body awareness, learn to release muscular tension and calm the mind. Yoga also promotes better sleep, which is crucial for caregivers who work shifting hours and often suffer from sleep disorders.

Integrating visualization techniques can also be a valuable tool for managing stress. Visualization involves imagining a soothing place or situation, focusing on sensory details such as colors, sounds, smells and sensations. This technique creates a "mental escape" from stressful situations, offering a moment of rest and mental recuperation. For example, by visualizing a serene landscape such as a beach or forest, the caregiver can induce a state of calm that helps reduce the stress response.

Developing time management and organizational strategies is also essential to reducing stress. Good organization helps to reduce the feeling of overload and better manage priorities. Planning your day, breaking tasks down into smaller, more manageable steps, and taking regular breaks are all strategies that can help reduce day-to-day pressure. Effective time management frees up space for moments of relaxation and recuperation, essential for maintaining balance and preventing burnout.

Finally, social support plays a crucial role in stress management. Sharing your experiences with colleagues, friends or loved ones helps you feel supported and understood. Simply talking about your concerns can ease the burden of stress and offer new perspectives on the problems you face. Participating in discussion groups, support groups or social activities can strengthen this support network, providing spaces where you can recharge emotionally and find collective solutions to challenges.

∘ The importance of psychological support and discussion groups

The importance of psychological support and discussion groups in the healthcare environment cannot be underestimated, especially for professionals who are confronted daily with situations of intense stress, human suffering, and sometimes bereavement. Caregivers' work, while deeply rewarding, is also emotionally demanding and can, in the long term, lead to feelings of fatigue, exhaustion and even burn-out. In this context, psychological support and participation in discussion groups offer valuable resources for preserving caregivers' mental health, strengthening their resilience and enabling them to continue to exercise their profession with compassion and efficiency.

Psychological support, whether individual or collective, is essential to help caregivers deal with the complex and often intense emotions they may experience in the course of their work. Whether managing patients' pain, providing end-of-life care or dealing with emergency situations, these experiences can leave deep emotional scars. Psychological support offers a safe space where caregivers can express their feelings, frustrations and concerns without fear of judgment. Talking about these experiences with a trained psychologist or counselor helps them to unburden themselves of the emotional burden they may be carrying, to find constructive ways of coping with stress, and to develop strategies for dealing with future challenges.

As a complement to individual psychological support, discussion groups bring a collective dimension that is particularly beneficial. These groups bring together caregivers facing similar professional realities, offering them a space to share their experiences, emotions and coping strategies. Participating in a discussion group helps to break down the isolation one can feel, especially when overwhelmed by professional responsibilities and complex emotions. Hearing the stories of colleagues and sharing one's own experiences fosters a sense of solidarity and belonging, reminding participants that they are not alone in facing these challenges.

Talking groups are also an opportunity to learn from others. Each caregiver brings with them personal strategies for dealing with stress, anxiety or bereavement. By sharing these strategies, group members enrich their own psychological toolbox, discovering new ways of overcoming difficulties. What's more, mutual support in a talk group strengthens collective resilience: together, caregivers can find solutions to the problems they encounter, whether professional or personal challenges.

The simple act of talking, of expressing feelings that we often keep to ourselves for fear of appearing vulnerable, is in itself a therapeutic act. Talking groups offer a space where speech is free, and where everyone can feel listened to and understood. This dynamic helps to release repressed emotions, reduce stress and anxiety, and restore a sense of control over one's professional and personal life. Validation of feelings by peers also plays a crucial role: knowing that others have gone through similar experiences and understand what you're feeling brings immense comfort.

Psychological support and discussion groups also help prevent burnout. Burn-out is often the result of accumulated stress, a feeling of powerlessness in the face of repetitive situations, and a lack of adequate support. By offering a regular space to talk and be listened to, these resources help identify the warning signs of burnout and intervene before the situation becomes critical. Sharing positive experiences and successes in a discussion group can also restore meaning to the work, reminding caregivers why they chose this profession and enabling them to reconnect with their initial motivation.

Finally, it's important to stress that psychological support and discussion groups are not just crisis interventions, but should be seen as ongoing prevention tools. Integrating these practices into caregivers' routines, and encouraging them to participate regularly, helps to maintain lasting psychological well-being. Healthcare establishments play a key role in facilitating access to these resources, integrating them into staff well-being policies, and creating a culture where the care of caregivers is as much a priority as that of patients.

- **Preventing burn-out**
  ◦ **Warning signs of burn-out**

Burn-out, or professional exhaustion, is an increasingly recognized phenomenon in the workplace, particularly in healthcare professions where emotional, physical and psychological demands are particularly high. Burn-out doesn't happen overnight; it sets in gradually, often insidiously, through a series of warning signs which, if left unrecognized and untreated, can lead to a significant deterioration in health and well-being. Identifying these signs early is essential to intervene in time and prevent the devastating effects of burn-out.

One of the first warning signs of burn-out is persistent, intense fatigue. This fatigue goes beyond the simple feeling of being tired after a long day's work; it is chronic and does not go away even after a night's sleep or a weekend's rest. People on the verge of burn-out may wake up in the morning already exhausted, without the energy to face the day. This fatigue can be accompanied by sleep disturbances, such as difficulty in falling asleep, frequent awakenings, or a feeling of non-restorative sleep, which only aggravate the feeling of exhaustion.

Another telltale sign is diminished commitment and motivation at work. What was once exciting or motivating may suddenly seem insurmountable or irrelevant. Caregivers may begin to feel a growing disinterest in their daily tasks, a loss of pleasure in their work, or a sense of emotional detachment. This disengagement may manifest itself in reduced productivity, frequent lateness, or a tendency to procrastinate on important tasks. This loss of motivation is often accompanied by a feeling of cynicism or negativity towards work, colleagues or even patients.

Emotional disorders are also important warning signs of burn-out. People on the verge of burn-out may become more irritable, impatient or prone to fits of anger. They may feel overwhelmed by tasks that once seemed manageable, and react disproportionately to stressful situations. Feelings of anxiety, sadness or despair may also become more frequent. In some cases, these emotional disorders can lead to depressive symptoms, such as loss of interest in daily activities, feelings of worthlessness or guilt, and persistent negative thoughts.

Physical signs should not be overlooked. The chronic stress associated with burn-out can lead to a series of somatic symptoms, such as frequent headaches, muscle aches, gastrointestinal problems or heart palpitations. These physical symptoms often reflect mental and emotional exhaustion, and can become disabling if left untreated. Under prolonged stress, the body can react with constant muscular tension, generalized fatigue, and increased vulnerability to infection and disease.

Burn-out can also manifest itself through changes in behavior and habits. For example, a burned-out person may begin to isolate him/herself socially, avoiding interactions with colleagues, friends or family. They may also adopt avoidance behaviors, such as shirking work responsibilities or refusing to make decisions. Increased use of substances, such as alcohol, tobacco or medication, can also be a warning sign, as these substances are sometimes used as a means of coping with increasing stress or anxiety.

Another warning sign to watch out for is loss of performance at work. Despite best efforts, a burned-out person may find it increasingly difficult to perform tasks effectively. They may make mistakes, have difficulty concentrating, and experience a loss of creativity or problem-solving ability. This drop in performance, combined with a feeling of frustration or shame, can lead to a vicious circle where stress and exhaustion intensify even further.

Finally, a persistent feeling of hopelessness or pessimism can be an early sign of burn-out. When you feel that nothing you do seems good enough, that your efforts go unrecognized, or that the future looks bleak and hopeless, it's crucial to recognize these feelings as warning signs. This feeling of hopelessness can lead to total disengagement from work, or even severe depression if no intervention is put in place.

∘   **Resources and support to prevent burnout**
Preventing burnout, particularly in professions as demanding as caregiving, is crucial to ensuring not only the health and well-being of individuals, but also the quality of care provided to patients. Burn-out is an insidious process that sets in gradually, often under the combined effect of chronic stress, work overload and lack of support. To prevent it, it is essential to put in place a set of resources and support adapted to the situation, enabling caregivers to maintain their physical and mental balance, recharge their batteries on a regular basis, and find solutions to the difficulties they encounter in their day-to-day practice.

One of the most important resources for preventing burnout is access to appropriate psychological support. This support can take the form of individual consultations with a psychologist or specialized counselor, who offers a safe space to express feelings, frustrations and concerns. Psychological support helps identify sources of stress, understand the mechanisms that lead to burnout, and develop personal strategies to better manage day-to-day challenges. This type of support is particularly useful for preventing the build-up of tension and learning to recognize the warning signs of burn-out before it's too late.

Training and awareness programs also play a key role in preventing burnout. These programs can include workshops on stress management, caring communication, time management and work-life balance. By taking part in these training courses, caregivers acquire concrete tools to better organize their work, learn to delegate where possible, and introduce relaxation practices into their daily routine. These skills are not only useful for preventing burnout, they also help to improve efficiency and job satisfaction, by enabling them to better manage the pressures inherent in the profession.

Peer support is another valuable resource for preventing burnout. Talking groups, regular team meetings and informal exchange spaces enable caregivers to share their experiences, support each other and create a culture of solidarity within the team. These moments of sharing strengthen the bonds between colleagues, create a sense of belonging and make them feel less isolated in the face of difficulties. Peer support is particularly important in times of intense stress, when the simple knowledge that you're not alone in going through a difficult period can provide extra comfort and motivation.

Work-life balance is another crucial factor in preventing burnout. Caregivers should be encouraged to preserve spaces for disconnection, where they can recharge their batteries outside of work. This can include leisure activities, family time, sport, or any other activity that brings pleasure and relaxation. Healthcare facilities can support this balance by ensuring that working hours are reasonable, offering opportunities for time off to rest and regenerate, and valuing taking time for oneself as an essential element of caregivers' health and well-being.

Institutional support is also crucial. Healthcare establishments have a key role to play in preventing burnout by implementing human resources management policies that take caregivers' needs into account. This can include reducing excessive workloads, implementing balanced team rotations, recognizing work accomplished, and offering ongoing training for professional development. A corporate culture that values employee well-being and encourages open dialogue about the challenges faced by caregivers is essential to creating a working environment where burnout is less likely to take hold.

Integrating relaxation and stress management techniques into caregivers' daily routines is another important strategy. Techniques such as mindfulness meditation, deep breathing, yoga, or progressive muscle relaxation can help reduce stress levels, improve sleep quality and build resilience in the face of work pressures. These practices, when encouraged and supported by the institution, become powerful tools for maintaining mental and emotional balance, even in demanding work environments.

Finally, preventing burnout also involves encouraging regular self-assessment of well-being. Caregivers must be encouraged to take regular stock of their emotional and physical state, to identify signs of excessive fatigue, loss of motivation or disengagement, and not to hesitate to ask for help when necessary. Recognizing personal limits and knowing when to rest or ask for support are essential skills for preventing long-term burnout.

In conclusion, preventing burnout requires a range of resources and support tailored to the specific needs of caregivers. These include psychological support, training, peer support, work-life balance, institutional support, and the integration of relaxation techniques. By implementing these strategies, healthcare organizations can not only prevent burnout, but also create a working environment where caregivers can thrive, remain motivated and continue to deliver quality care with the empathy and commitment that characterize their profession.

Chapter 9

The Night Care Aide and Technological Innovations

- **The evolution of night-time care technologies**
  - **Remote monitoring devices and their impact**

Remote monitoring devices have revolutionized the way care is delivered, offering innovative solutions to improve the quality of care, enhance patient safety, and optimize the work of caregivers. These technologies, which enable real-time monitoring of patients' state of health without the need to be physically present at their side, are having a significant impact on medical practice, particularly in environments where human resources are limited or the need for continuous monitoring is high.

One of the main advantages of remote monitoring devices is their ability to provide constant vigilance. These systems, whether vital signs monitors, motion sensors or connected wearable devices, enable continuous monitoring of essential parameters such as heart rate, oxygen saturation, blood pressure and body temperature. In real time, this data is transmitted to a central interface where caregivers can consult it instantly. This continuous monitoring is particularly valuable in intensive care units, neonatology wards, or at home for at-risk patients. It enables the rapid detection of any anomaly, anticipating complications and reacting before the situation becomes critical.

These devices also reduce caregivers' workload by automating monitoring tasks that would otherwise require a constant presence at the bedside. In an environment where staff are often under pressure and staffing levels can be reduced, the ability to monitor multiple patients simultaneously, even remotely, frees up time for caregivers. This means they can concentrate on other aspects of their work, such as direct patient care, accompanying patients, or managing medical records. This contributes to a better distribution of tasks and more efficient use of available human resources.

The integration of these remote monitoring technologies also enhances patient safety. By detecting signs of deterioration at an early stage, such as a sudden drop in oxygen saturation or a rapid increase in heart rate, the devices enable rapid intervention that can prevent serious outcomes. This enhanced reactivity is particularly beneficial for patients with chronic or complex pathologies, for whom close monitoring is essential to avoid frequent hospitalization or severe complications.

In addition, remote monitoring devices promote the autonomy of patients, particularly those suffering from chronic illnesses or the elderly. By enabling them to stay at home while being monitored remotely, these technologies reduce the need for frequent hospital visits, thus reducing the stress and inconvenience associated with travel. Patients often feel more comfortable and secure in their own homes, while having the peace of mind that their condition is being closely monitored. This not only improves their quality of life, but also their adherence to treatment, as they feel supported and cared for, even at a distance.

However, the impact of remote monitoring devices is not limited to purely technical or clinical aspects. They are also transforming the relationship between patients and caregivers. The ability to collect data in real time creates a new dynamic in care, where the caregiver becomes a companion who, thanks to the data, can personalize interventions and advice. This personalization of care boosts patient confidence and improves the quality of interactions, even if they take place at a distance. By being constantly informed of their patients' condition, caregivers can adapt their approach more precisely and proactively, enhancing the effectiveness of care.

However, these devices also pose challenges, particularly in terms of data management and security. The massive collection of often sensitive healthcare data requires robust protection systems to guarantee confidentiality and prevent the risk of cyber-attacks. Healthcare establishments must therefore invest in secure infrastructures and train their staff in the management of these technologies to avoid any malfunctions or data leaks.

In terms of psychological impact, it's important to recognize that the use of remote monitoring devices can also have ambivalent effects. For some patients, knowing that they are being constantly monitored can bring peace of mind. However, for others, it can generate a sense of loss of control or dependency, or even intrusion into their private lives. It is therefore essential that the introduction of these technologies is accompanied by clear, empathetic communication, explaining the benefits, but also respecting patients' preferences and comfort.

Finally, the evolution of remote monitoring devices has important implications for caregiver training. Healthcare professionals need to be trained not only in the technical use of these devices, but also in the interpretation of the data they generate. They need to be able to make clinical decisions based on the information provided by these technologies, while maintaining a human, patient-centered approach.

- ◦ **Real-time use of electronic medical records (EMRs)**

The use of real-time electronic medical records (EMRs) has profoundly transformed the healthcare landscape, offering a multitude of benefits that improve both the efficiency of care and the quality of patient management. By centralizing and instantly updating medical information, these digital tools provide caregivers with a complete and up-to-date view of patients' health status, enabling faster, more informed and better coordinated decision-making.

One of the key benefits of real-time EMRs is their ability to provide healthcare professionals with immediate, secure access to a patient's medical data, regardless of their location. This accessibility is crucial, especially in emergency situations where every second counts. Caregivers can consult medical histories, test results, prescriptions and clinical notes in just a few clicks, without having to search for paper files or wait for information to be transmitted from one department to another. This rapid access improves not only responsiveness to critical situations, but also continuity of care, by ensuring that every intervention is informed by the most up-to-date data.

Real-time EMRs also facilitate coordination between the various healthcare professionals involved in a patient's care. In a hospital environment, where several specialists, nurses and technicians may intervene on the same case, the EMR ensures that everyone has the same information at the same time. This reduces the risk of errors, such as duplicate tests or unwanted drug interactions, and ensures that everyone is aligned with the same care plan. This increased coordination contributes to more coherent and efficient care, reducing wasted time and misunderstandings.

Another significant advantage of real-time EMRs is the ability to integrate automated alerts and reminders into the care process. For example, the EMR can flag an anomaly in a test result, remind the patient of a due vaccination, or warn of a potential drug interaction. These proactive features help caregivers to avoid missing important information, and to intervene preventively rather than reactively. What's more, these alerts can be tailored to the specific needs of each patient, enabling truly individualized care.

EMRs also play a crucial role in improving the quality of care, thanks to the traceability and transparency they offer. Every modification to the file, every intervention, every decision is recorded, creating a complete and detailed history of the patient's care. This traceability is essential not only to ensure continuity of care, but also to evaluate medical practices, conduct quality audits, and identify areas for improvement. By having a precise, chronological record of all actions and observations, healthcare facilities can better understand care trajectories and implement strategies to optimize patient outcomes.

Data security is another key aspect of using real-time EMRs. Modern EMR systems are designed to protect sensitive information through advanced security protocols, such as data encryption and user authentication. These measures ensure that only authorized persons can access medical records, protecting patient confidentiality while facilitating safe and efficient information sharing. In a context where the protection of personal data is increasingly regulated, EMRs offer a solution that complies with legal requirements while meeting the operational needs of caregivers.

In terms of practicality, real-time EMRs offer unprecedented flexibility in care management. Caregivers can access patient records from any connected device - computer, tablet or smartphone - anywhere. This accessibility enables greater mobility for healthcare professionals, who can consult or update records while on the move within the facility, or even remotely, during teleconsultations for example. This flexibility translates into better time management and reduced delays between decision-making and intervention.

However, the adoption of real-time EMRs is not without its challenges. It is crucial that caregivers are trained in the use of these systems to take full advantage of them. A poorly designed user interface or poor integration into existing workflows can lead to frustration and errors. It is therefore essential that healthcare facilities invest in intuitive, ergonomic EMR systems, accompanied by appropriate training programs that enable users to quickly familiarize themselves with the new technologies.

- **New tools for the night orderly**
  - **Mobile applications and digital tools for care management**

Mobile applications and digital tools have taken on an increasingly important role in care management, offering healthcare professionals innovative ways to improve the quality, efficiency and accessibility of the services they provide. These technologies, which range from patient tracking applications to team communication tools, are transforming the way care is organized and delivered, facilitating coordination, optimizing processes and increasing responsiveness to patient needs.

One of the main contributions of mobile applications to care management is to improve communication and coordination between different members of the healthcare team. Secure messaging applications enable doctors, nurses and other healthcare professionals to share information in real time, exchange medical opinions, and coordinate interventions seamlessly, while respecting data confidentiality. This is particularly crucial in environments where the speed of communication can have a direct impact on treatment decisions and patient outcomes. For example, when a patient presents critical symptoms, the ability to quickly consult a specialist via a mobile app can speed up decision-making and potentially save lives.

Digital tools have also transformed patient monitoring, both in hospitals and at home. Apps for tracking vital vitals, managing medication, or monitoring symptoms enable caregivers to collect and analyze data in real time. This information, often gathered from connected devices such as smartwatches or medical sensors, is then accessible via digital platforms, where it can be reviewed by healthcare professionals. This continuous, remote monitoring is particularly beneficial for patients suffering from chronic illnesses, who require regular monitoring but can avoid frequent hospitalization thanks to these tools. Automatic alerts, should any anomalies be detected, enable rapid intervention before the situation becomes critical.

Mobile applications also facilitate patient education and empowerment. Many apps are designed to help patients better understand their condition, follow their treatment, keep medical appointments, and adopt positive health behaviors. For example, a diabetes management app can help a patient track their blood sugar levels, adjust their diet accordingly, and remember to take their medication on time. By involving patients in their own care,

157

these digital tools promote better treatment adherence and increased engagement in their care pathway.

Administrative efficiency is another area where digital tools are having a significant impact. Care management applications facilitate appointment scheduling, medical record management, billing and patient communication. These tools reduce the time spent on administrative tasks, freeing caregivers to concentrate more on direct care. For example, an online appointment scheduling application can reduce phone calls and scheduling errors, while a digital records management system simplifies access to and updating of medical information, reducing the risk of errors and redundancies.

Digital tools also offer opportunities for continuing education and knowledge sharing for healthcare professionals. Applications and educational platforms enable caregivers to keep abreast of the latest medical advances, take part in online courses, and collaborate with colleagues around the world. These digital resources enrich caregivers' expertise and contribute to the continuous improvement of care quality. For example, a training application can offer modules on new surgical techniques or emergency management, accessible at any time and from any location, facilitating ongoing professional development.

However, the adoption of mobile applications and digital tools in care management is not without its challenges. It is essential to ensure that these technologies are intuitive, accessible and well integrated into existing work processes. Poor design or inadequate use can lead to frustration, errors or even risks to patient safety. In addition, staff training in the use of these technologies is crucial to ensure that they are used optimally and deliver the expected benefits. Data security is another critical aspect, as healthcare information is particularly sensitive. Applications must therefore comply with strict data protection standards to ensure that patient confidentiality is preserved.

◦ Artificial intelligence and its role in monitoring patients at night

Artificial intelligence (AI) is playing an increasingly crucial role in healthcare, particularly when it comes to monitoring patients at night, a time when vigilance and continuous surveillance are particularly necessary, but when human resources can be limited. Integrating AI into night-time patient monitoring offers innovative solutions to improve care safety, detect signs of deterioration early and lighten the workload of caregivers, enabling them to focus on higher value-added tasks.

One of the most promising applications of AI in night-time monitoring is real-time vital signs monitoring. AI systems are capable of continuously analyzing data collected by connected medical devices, such as heart rate, oxygen saturation, or blood pressure monitors. Thanks to sophisticated algorithms, these systems can identify subtle trends or anomalies that might go unnoticed by the human eye, especially during the hours of the night when fatigue can affect caregivers' vigilance. For example, a slight increase in heart rate or a gradual drop in oxygenation could be interpreted by the AI as an early sign of a complication, triggering an alert for rapid intervention before the situation becomes critical.

AI not only detects anomalies, it also learns from the accumulated data, becoming increasingly accurate in its predictions over time. This type of machine learning enables AI systems to adapt to the specifics of each patient, offering personalized monitoring that takes into account medical history, current treatments, and specific physiological responses. This ability to adapt is particularly valuable for patients with chronic diseases or those in critical states, where subtle changes can have far-reaching implications.

In addition to monitoring vital signs, AI also plays a key role in alarm management. In a hospital environment, particularly at night, alarms can be frequent, sometimes due to false alarms or minor anomalies. Alarm overload, known as "alarm fatigue", can cause caregivers to become desensitized, increasing the risk of missing a critical alert. AI systems can help filter alarms by analyzing contextual data and prioritizing alerts according to their actual severity. For example, AI can differentiate between an alarm triggered by a poorly positioned sensor and one indicating a real deterioration in the patient's condition, thus reducing the number of false alarms and improving caregivers' responsiveness.

AI also contributes to night-time care planning by optimizing resource allocation. By analyzing data from several patients at the same time, AI can identify those requiring increased monitoring and adjust the allocation of tasks among available caregivers accordingly. This ensures that resources are concentrated where they are most needed, while easing the workload on caregivers so they can concentrate on direct care. This optimization is particularly important at night, when shifts are often small and each team member has multiple responsibilities to manage.

Artificial intelligence also improves communication between care teams, particularly in the handover of services between day and night. AI systems can synthesize information gathered during the night and provide a concise but comprehensive report to daytime teams, highlighting critical points and necessary actions. This continuity in communication ensures that care is seamless, and that transitions between teams are seamless, with no loss of important information.

Finally, the use of AI in patient monitoring at night also contributes to improved well-being for caregivers. By automating certain monitoring tasks and reducing the number of false alarms, AI can reduce the stress and cognitive load on caregivers, offering them a more serene working environment. This can also lead to a reduction in the risk of burnout, by enabling caregivers to focus on the more rewarding aspects of their work, such as patient interaction and direct care.

However, despite its many advantages, the integration of AI into nocturnal patient monitoring needs to be approached with caution.

It is essential that caregivers are trained in the use of these technologies, that they understand how AI systems make decisions, and that they are able to intervene when necessary. AI must be seen as a complementary tool that supports the work of caregivers, not as a replacement for human expertise. Trust in these systems is crucial, and this can only be achieved through a combination of training, transparency and collaboration between technology and caregivers.

- **Challenges and opportunities linked to the adoption of new technologies**
  - ◦ **Adapting to new technologies: training and updating skills**

Adapting to new technologies has become an inescapable necessity in the healthcare field, where technological innovations are rapidly transforming practices, tools and working methods. This constant evolution requires healthcare professionals to undergo continuous training and regularly update their skills to remain at the cutting edge of their field. Training and skills updating are no longer options, but imperatives to guarantee safe, effective, quality care.

New technologies, whether electronic medical records (EMRs), remote monitoring devices, mobile applications or artificial intelligence, offer incredible possibilities for improving patient care. However, their successful adoption largely depends on caregivers' ability to understand them, use them effectively, and integrate them seamlessly into their daily practice. This is where training plays a crucial role. Well-designed initial training enables healthcare professionals to familiarize themselves with the new tools, understand how they work and what they can be used for, and acquire the skills they need to use them with confidence.

Training must be continuous, because technologies evolve rapidly, and what is innovative today may be obsolete tomorrow.

Ongoing training programs enable caregivers to keep abreast of the latest advances, adapt their skills to new requirements, and avoid being overwhelmed by the speed of change. These programs need to be flexible, accessible and adapted to the specific needs of healthcare professionals, taking into account their often restrictive work schedules. Online training, interactive webinars and hands-on workshops are particularly effective formats for offering this flexibility, while ensuring that skills are regularly updated.

Adapting to new technologies is more than just learning the ropes. It also involves understanding the ethical, legal and practical implications of these tools. For example, the use of EMRs or AI in patient care raises important questions about data confidentiality, system security, and the relationship between caregiver and patient. Training courses must therefore include modules on these aspects to prepare caregivers to face these challenges and use technologies responsibly.

Another crucial aspect of adapting to new technologies is the ability to integrate these tools into existing workflows. Caregivers must learn not only how to use new technologies, but also how to integrate them seamlessly into their daily routine without disrupting patient care. This may require adjustments to time management, task allocation and communication within the care team. Training courses must therefore include practical scenarios and simulations that enable caregivers to practice integrating these tools into real-life situations, in order to minimize disruptions and optimize their use.

Institutional support is also essential to facilitate this adaptation. Healthcare establishments must invest in quality training programs, offer easy access to continuing education resources, and encourage a culture of lifelong learning. They must also recognize the importance of updating skills, and reward caregivers' efforts to train and adapt. This can take the form of incentives, formal recognition or career development opportunities for those who demonstrate a commitment to continuous skills improvement.

Collaboration between healthcare professionals and technology developers is another important dimension of this adaptation. Caregivers need to be involved in the development and implementation of new technologies, as their feedback is crucial to designing tools that truly meet the needs of the field. This collaboration can take the form of working groups, advisory committees or partnerships with technology companies. By being part of the process, caregivers can ensure that technologies are not only innovative, but also practical, intuitive and genuinely useful in their day-to-day work.

Finally, adapting to new technologies should be seen not as a burden, but as an opportunity. An opportunity to modernize practices, improve care efficiency, reduce errors, and deliver a better patient experience. Caregivers who embrace this evolution with a positive attitude and a willingness to learn will not only continue to excel in their profession, but also play a key role in the future of healthcare. Technologies are powerful tools which, when used correctly, can free up time for caregivers, enabling them to focus more on the human aspects of their work, such as empathy, listening, and accompanying patients.

○   **Assessing the impact of technology on quality of care and staff well-being**

Assessing the impact of technology on the quality of care and well-being of healthcare staff has become a central issue in the current context of digital transformation of healthcare systems. Technological innovations such as electronic medical records, remote monitoring devices and communication tools have the potential to revolutionize medical practice. However, their adoption raises crucial questions: do these technologies really improve the quality of care delivered to patients? And what is their effect on the well-being of caregivers, who have to juggle the use of these tools with their daily tasks?

One of the main aims of healthcare technologies is to improve the quality of care. To assess this impact, it is essential to look at a number of indicators, such as patient safety, treatment effectiveness and patient satisfaction. Technologies can contribute to better patient care by enabling more accurate monitoring, more efficient data management, and more informed decision-making. For example, electronic medical records facilitate rapid access to a patient's medical history, reducing the risk of medication errors or misdiagnoses. Similarly, remote monitoring systems enable signs of deterioration to be detected earlier, which can lead to faster interventions and potentially save lives.

However, for these benefits to be realized, it is crucial that technologies are well integrated into care practices. This means they must be user-friendly, intuitive, and adapted to the specific needs of healthcare professionals. Poorly designed or overly complex tools can lead to errors, frustration and resistance to adoption, which can ultimately harm the quality of care. It is therefore important to evaluate not only clinical outcomes, but also the user experience of caregivers to ensure that technologies enhance rather than hinder their work.

Assessing the impact of technologies on staff well-being is equally crucial. Caregivers are often faced with intense workloads and high levels of stress, and the introduction of new technologies can either alleviate or exacerbate these pressures. On the one hand, technologies can simplify certain tasks, automate repetitive processes, and enable better time management, freeing caregivers to concentrate on higher value-added activities, such as direct patient care. For example, a care management application can reduce the time spent on administrative tasks, enabling nurses to devote more time to listening to and supporting patients.

On the other hand, if technologies are not well adapted, or if carers are not sufficiently trained in their use, they can add to mental load and stress. The phenomenon of "digital fatigue", where carers feel overwhelmed by the need to manage multiple digital systems in parallel, is an example of how technology can sometimes complicate rather than facilitate work. What's more, the demand for constant availability via communication tools can blur the boundaries between professional and personal life, contributing to burnout.

To properly assess the impact of technologies on staff well-being, it is necessary to consider several dimensions, including workload, job satisfaction, and work-life balance. Satisfaction surveys, interviews with caregivers, and field observation studies can provide valuable insights into how technologies are perceived and experienced by those who use them on a daily basis. These assessments should be carried out regularly to adjust tools and practices in response to staff feedback.

Another important aspect to consider is change management. The introduction of new technologies often requires a period of adaptation, during which caregivers must learn to master new tools while continuing to provide quality care. Adequate support in the form of training, mentoring and technical assistance is essential to minimize disruption and maximize the benefits of technology. In addition, involving caregivers in the technology selection and implementation process can increase their acceptance and commitment, as they then feel part of the changes affecting their practice.

Finally, technology impact assessment must include long-term thinking. The benefits of technologies may not be immediately apparent, and some negative effects may only become apparent after an extended period of use. It is therefore important to carry out longitudinal evaluations, tracking the evolution of indicators of care quality and staff well-being over several years. These long-term studies enable us to better understand the cumulative effects of technologies, and to make informed decisions on whether to maintain, modify or replace them.

Chapter 10

Medication management on the night shift

- **The caregiver's responsibilities in medication management**
  ◦ **Treatment administration: protocol compliance and safety**

Administering treatment to patients is one of the most critical responsibilities in healthcare. It demands absolute rigor to guarantee patient safety and effective care. Adherence to protocols and safety in the administration of treatment are fundamental pillars that ensure not only the proper execution of care, but also patient confidence in the healthcare system. Even the slightest error in drug administration can have serious consequences, ranging from treatment ineffectiveness to potentially fatal side effects. That's why precision, vigilance and scrupulous adherence to protocols are essential.

Treatment protocols are sets of standardized instructions designed to guide healthcare professionals in the administration of drugs. These protocols take into account best practices, scientific recommendations, specific patient characteristics and possible drug interactions. Strict adherence to them considerably reduces the risk of medication errors, which can occur at various stages, from prescribing to preparation and administration. Protocols detail precise doses, modes of administration, schedules and contraindications, ensuring that each patient receives the appropriate treatment, tailored to his or her specific state of health.

Ongoing training of caregivers is crucial to ensure compliance with these protocols. Drugs and technologies are constantly evolving, and it is essential that caregivers are regularly informed of new recommendations, changes to existing protocols, and the introduction of new drugs. Training also raises staff awareness of common errors and how to avoid them, reinforcing a safety culture where every team member is aware of the importance of their role in the care chain. Training sessions, hands-on workshops and access to educational resources are all ways of maintaining a high level of competence among caregivers.

The use of technologies such as computerized prescribing systems and electronic medical records (EMRs) also plays a key role in ensuring compliance with protocols and the safe administration of treatments. These digital tools can centralize patient information, check prescriptions in real time, and automatically detect potentially dangerous drug interactions. For example, an electronic prescription system can immediately alert a caregiver if a prescribed dose exceeds the safe limit, or if a drug is incompatible with another treatment in progress. These systems reduce the risk of human error and ensure double-checking, which reinforces the safety of care.

Communication between members of the healthcare team is another essential element in guaranteeing safety when administering treatments. Good communication ensures that all professionals involved in a patient's care are aware of current treatments, any changes, and specific precautions to be taken. Communication between teams, whether during shift changes or between different departments, must be clear, complete and precise, to avoid any confusion or omissions. Regular meetings to discuss complex cases, difficulties encountered, and measures to be taken, reinforce this communication and enable any deviations from protocols to be quickly corrected.

Adherence to protocols should not be seen as a mere bureaucratic obligation, but as an essential component of quality care. Each protocol is the fruit of in-depth research and long clinical experience, aimed at standardizing best practices to offer each patient the safest and most effective treatment. For caregivers, following a protocol means not only administering a drug, but also ensuring that all stages of care are carried out to the same high standard, from checking prescriptions to monitoring the effects of treatment.

It's also important to recognize that adherence to protocols must be accompanied by constant vigilance and the ability to react quickly to problems. Sometimes, unforeseen situations may arise, requiring adaptation of protocols. In such cases, caregivers must be able to assess the situation, make informed decisions, and document these adjustments to ensure continuity and safety of care. This flexibility, when supported by a sound knowledge of protocols and effective communication, enables a high level of safety to be maintained while meeting the specific needs of patients.

○ The importance of traceability and transmission during team changes

Traceability and communication during team changes are crucial to guaranteeing continuity and quality of care in healthcare establishments. These processes ensure that every patient receives consistent, uninterrupted care, even when care teams change. The importance of traceability and transmission cannot be underestimated, as they play a central role in preventing errors, improving communication between healthcare professionals, and making care safer.

The traceability of medical acts and care is essential to document every stage of a patient's care. It involves systematically recording in detail all interventions, clinical observations, treatments administered and decisions taken. These records enable us to retrace the complete history of the care received by the patient, providing a clear and precise frame of reference for the caregivers who take over when the team changes. Rigorous traceability ensures that nothing is left to chance, and that all relevant information is available in real time to guide clinical decisions.

Traceability plays a fundamental role in inter-team communications, providing a reliable, structured source of information. Transmissions involve an exchange of information between current and future caregivers. They must be precise, complete and carried out in clear language to avoid any confusion or misunderstanding. Effective transmission relies on the ability to communicate the essential information concisely, while ensuring that critical details are not overlooked. This includes the patient's current clinical status, ongoing treatments, recent observations, any complications, and priorities for the next team. A well-maintained traceability file greatly facilitates these transmissions by providing rapid access to all the necessary information.

The importance of transmission is accentuated in contexts where patients have complex needs or are in critical condition. In these situations, any omission or inaccuracy in a transmission can have serious, even life-threatening, consequences. For example, if a change in a patient's condition is not properly communicated, the new team may not react in time, or may make inappropriate decisions. So, rigorous, well-structured transmission is essential to ensure that every caregiver has the information they need to act appropriately right from the start of their shift.

Traceability and communication also help to reinforce collective responsibility within care teams. By ensuring accurate documentation and effective communication, each caregiver contributes to the quality and safety of care. This shared responsibility creates a culture of trust, where each team member knows he or she can rely on the rigor and professionalism of colleagues. This reduces stress and uncertainty during transitions, and fosters better collaboration between teams, which is particularly important in high-pressure work environments such as intensive care units or emergency departments.

The implementation of standardized protocols for transmissions and traceability is another key factor in their effectiveness. These protocols provide a clear framework for what is to be communicated and how it is to be done. They can include checklists to ensure that all important points are covered, standardized reporting formats for ease of reading and understanding, and double-checking systems to guarantee the accuracy of information. The use of digital technologies, such as electronic medical records, can also improve the quality of transmissions by enabling instant, centralized access to all relevant data.

However, traceability and transmission should not be seen as mere administrative formalities. Above all, they are essential clinical practices that contribute directly to the quality of care. It is important that caregivers understand their value and approach them with the same level of rigor as other aspects of their clinical work. Training and ongoing awareness of the importance of traceability and transmissions must be an integral part of caregivers' professional development, to reinforce their commitment to these crucial practices.

- **Risks associated with night-time medication management**
  - **Preventing medication errors in fatigue situations**

Preventing medication errors in situations of fatigue is a major challenge in healthcare. Fatigue, particularly among caregivers, is a well-documented risk factor that can lead to reduced vigilance, errors in judgment, and a diminished ability to perform complex tasks with precision. In an environment where medication errors can have serious, even fatal, consequences, it is crucial to put in place effective strategies to minimize risk, even when caregivers are fatigued.

The first step in preventing medication errors in situations of fatigue is to recognize fatigue itself as a significant risk. Healthcare facilities need to foster a culture where caregivers are aware of the signs of fatigue and can report them without fear of stigmatization. Fatigue can manifest itself in a variety of ways: drowsiness, difficulty concentrating, irritability, or even slowed reflexes. These signs need to be taken seriously, as they can impair the caregiver's ability to follow protocols rigorously.

To counter the effects of fatigue, reinforced safety protocols are essential. Double-check systems are one of the most effective ways of preventing medication errors. When a caregiver prepares a medication, another person must check the dose, the route of administration, the patient's name, and the medication itself. This double check can detect potential errors before they occur, providing an extra layer of safety. This process is particularly crucial during periods of high fatigue, when typing or reading errors are more likely.

The use of digital technologies, such as electronic prescribing systems, also helps to reduce medication errors. These systems are designed to automate certain tasks, such as calculating doses or checking for drug interactions, thereby reducing the cognitive load on caregivers. By integrating automatic alerts that signal unusual doses or contraindications, these technologies can act as safeguards, reminding caregivers to double-check before administering a drug. However, it is important that caregivers are well trained in the use of these technologies to avoid over-reliance or blind trust in them, which could paradoxically lead to errors if the systems are misused or fail.

Managing working hours is another crucial lever for preventing fatigue and, by extension, medication errors. Caregivers working long hours, especially those on night shifts, are more likely to make mistakes. It is therefore essential that healthcare establishments put in place policies that limit consecutive working hours and ensure that caregivers have sufficient rest time between shifts. Regular breaks during long shifts are also important to enable caregivers to rest and recuperate, even if only for a few minutes.

At the same time, ongoing training plays an essential role in preventing medication errors. Regular training sessions on good medication administration practices, managing stressful situations, and strategies for remaining vigilant despite fatigue are essential. Such training can include simulations of situations where fatigue is a factor, enabling caregivers to practice decision-making under pressure in a controlled environment. This helps them to better manage such situations in the real world, thus reducing the risk of errors.

Communication within care teams is also a key element in preventing medication errors in fatigue situations. Clear, open communication ensures that all team members are aware of current treatments, recent changes, and specific patient concerns. Encouraging caregivers to ask for help or point out any uncertainties can help prevent errors that might otherwise go unnoticed in a fatigued environment.

Finally, it's essential to create a working environment that supports caregivers' well-being. This includes not only managing schedules and providing adequate breaks, but also psychological support and access to resources to manage stress and fatigue. Workplace wellness programs, comfortable rest areas, and an organizational culture that values caregivers' mental health all help to reduce the risks associated with fatigue.

   ○   **Vigilance when administering sedative or opioid drugs**

Vigilance when administering sedative or opioid drugs is absolutely essential due to the high potential of these substances to cause serious, even fatal, adverse effects if not used with the utmost caution. Sedatives and opioids, while valuable for pain and anxiety management, present significant risks such as respiratory depression, excessive drowsiness and dependence. That's why every stage of their administration must be surrounded by rigorous measures to guarantee patient safety.

The crucial first step is a thorough assessment of the patient before these drugs are administered. This assessment includes not only a review of the patient's medical history, but also careful attention to his or her current conditions. Caregivers need to take into account factors such as age, weight, renal and liver function, and the presence of comorbidities, all of which can influence how the patient metabolizes these substances. For example, elderly

174

patients or those with renal failure may be more sensitive to the effects of opioids, requiring dose adjustments to avoid excessive sedation or toxicity.

Adherence to dosing protocols is another fundamental aspect of vigilance. Opioids and sedatives have narrow therapeutic windows, meaning that the margin between an effective dose and a dangerous one can be small. Caregivers must therefore scrupulously follow dosing recommendations and use appropriate measuring devices to ensure the accuracy of doses administered. This includes checking multiple doses and complying with institutional protocols, which often call for double-checking by a second caregiver, especially in the context of high doses or continuous infusions.

Continuous monitoring after the administration of sedatives or opioids is essential for early detection of signs of an adverse reaction. Respiratory depression, one of the most feared complications, requires particular attention. Caregivers must frequently monitor the patient's vital signs, in particular respiratory rate, oxygen saturation and consciousness. Cardiorespiratory monitors can be used to provide real-time surveillance, enabling immediate intervention in the event of deterioration. Constant communication with the patient is also essential to assess sedation levels and detect early signs of overdosage, such as unusual drowsiness or difficulty staying awake.

Adjusting doses according to patient response is another key aspect of vigilance. Caregivers must be prepared to modify doses according to the patient's tolerance to the drug, taking care not to exceed the maximum recommended doses. In some cases, the administration of an antagonist, such as naloxone for opioids, may be necessary to reverse the effects of sedation or accidental overdose. Knowing the indications and administration protocols for these antagonists is essential to react quickly when needed.

Vigilance in the administration of these drugs also implies rigorous documentation. Each administration of a sedative or opioid must be accurately recorded in the patient's medical record, including dose, route of administration, time of day and post-administration clinical observations. This documentation enables the patient's progress to be monitored, any abnormalities to be rapidly identified, and continuity of care to be guaranteed when there is a change of team. What's more, in the event of complications, precise documentation is essential for analyzing events and adjusting protocols if necessary.

Ongoing training of caregivers is another pillar of vigilance. Given the risks associated with these drugs, it is crucial that healthcare professionals are regularly trained in the latest practices and recommendations for the safe administration of sedatives and opioids. This includes training in the recognition of early signs of overdose, the management of side effects, and the use of monitoring devices. Critical situation simulations can also be an effective tool for preparing caregivers to respond appropriately in an emergency.

Finally, open and proactive communication with the patient is essential. Patients must be informed of the potential effects of sedatives or opioids, including the risks, and encouraged to report any unusual symptoms. This communication not only promotes vigilance on the part of the caregiver, but also on the part of the patient, who becomes an active partner in monitoring his or her own health.

In conclusion, vigilance when administering sedative or opioid drugs is a complex process requiring constant attention, close monitoring and effective communication. By combining rigorous pre-assessment, adherence to dosing protocols, continuous monitoring, accurate documentation and ongoing training, caregivers can minimize risks and ensure safe administration of these powerful drugs. This vigilance is essential to protect patients while offering them the therapeutic benefits necessary for their comfort and recovery.

- **The caregiver's role in observing the effects of medication**
  - **Monitoring patients' reactions after taking medication**

Monitoring patients' reactions after taking medication is a crucial step in the care process, ensuring both treatment efficacy and patient safety. Each patient may react differently to a drug, depending on a variety of factors, such as age, general health, medical history and other medications taken. Careful monitoring of post-medication reactions enables us not only to detect any adverse effects, but also to adjust treatment according to the patient's response, in order to optimize well-being and recovery.

The first phase of monitoring involves being vigilant as soon as the drug is administered. It is essential that the caregiver observes the patient immediately after administration to spot any abnormal reactions. The first minutes and hours after administration are often critical, especially for fast-acting drugs or those with a high allergic potential. Signs such as redness, itching, swelling, breathing difficulties, or a sudden change in blood pressure should be monitored closely, as they may indicate a severe allergic reaction, such as anaphylaxis, requiring immediate intervention.

Secondly, continuous monitoring of vital signs is essential. Medications can affect heart rate, blood pressure, breathing and body temperature. Regular monitoring of these parameters enables early detection of any significant changes that could signal a problem. For example, a drop in blood pressure or bradycardia (slowing of the heart rate) after the administration of a sedative drug should be reported immediately, as it may indicate an overdose or increased sensitivity of the patient to the drug.

At the same time, it's important to observe the patient's subjective reactions. Every patient is unique, and their personal feelings after taking a drug are a valuable indicator of treatment tolerance. Caregivers should encourage patients to express any discomfort, dizziness, nausea or other symptoms they feel, however minor they may seem. These subjective signs may reveal side effects that are not immediately apparent, but which may worsen if treatment is not adjusted. For example, persistent nausea after taking an antibiotic may indicate intolerance, or the need to change the route of administration.

Medium- and long-term monitoring of side effects is also crucial, especially for drugs taken over an extended period. Some side effects may take several days or weeks to appear, such as toxic accumulation of a substance, delayed immune response, or metabolic effects. Caregivers should therefore be alert to progressive changes in the patient's condition, such as the appearance of neurological symptoms, changes in liver or kidney function, or endocrine disorders. Regular clinical examinations and laboratory tests may be necessary to monitor these long-term effects, especially in the case of potentially toxic or complex treatments.

Communication with the healthcare team is another fundamental aspect of monitoring post-medication reactions. Caregivers must record all observations and reactions in detail in the patient's medical record. This information must be shared with the whole care team during transmissions, to ensure continuity of care and enable each team member to make informed decisions based on the patient's progress. Clear and precise communication avoids omissions and errors, ensuring that all caregivers involved are aware of the patient's particularities and the necessary adaptations to treatment.

Adjusting treatment in response to observed reactions is the last essential step in this monitoring process. If a patient presents signs of intolerance or significant side effects, it is often necessary to modify the dosage, change the drug, or adjust the route of administration. This decision must be taken in consultation with the prescribing physician, taking into account the patient's general condition and therapeutic objectives. For example, if a patient suffers severe side effects after taking an opioid for pain management, another less potent analgesic or a combination with an adjuvant could be considered to reduce the dose of opioid required while maintaining effective pain control.

◦ Reporting adverse events and adjusting care

Reporting adverse events and adjusting care are key elements in ensuring patient safety and the effectiveness of medical treatments. These two closely linked actions play a fundamental role in clinical management, enabling care to be rapidly adapted to individual patient reactions to drugs or therapeutic interventions.

Reporting adverse events is a crucial step in the therapeutic follow-up of patients. Adverse events, whether minor or serious, must be systematically observed, noted and reported by caregivers. Undesirable effects can manifest themselves in a variety of ways, from allergic reactions and unexpected side-effects to functional disorders and more serious complications such as organ damage. Early recognition of these effects can prevent more severe complications and ensure that treatment remains beneficial to the patient.

Caregivers' vigilance is essential in this process. Every member of the healthcare team must be trained to identify the potential signs of an adverse reaction, even when these are subtle or atypical. For example, mild pruritus or a rash following the administration of an antibiotic may be a precursor to a more serious allergic reaction, such as anaphylaxis. Similarly, signs such as persistent headaches, dizziness or gastrointestinal disturbances may indicate that the drug is not being tolerated by the patient, and require further evaluation.

Once an adverse reaction has been detected, it must be reported immediately. Reporting must be done in accordance with the protocols established within the healthcare establishment, often by recording observations in the patient's medical record and alerting the prescribing physician or multidisciplinary team concerned. This precise documentation includes a description of the adverse reaction, the time of onset, the dose of medication administered, and any other relevant information that may help to understand the patient's reaction. This reporting is not only a legal and ethical obligation, but also a valuable tool for adjusting care appropriately and contributing to pharmacovigilance, a post-marketing drug monitoring system.

Adjustment of care, following the reporting of an adverse event, is the immediate, proactive response to ensure patient safety. This adjustment can take many forms, depending on the severity of the adverse reaction and the patient's general condition. In some cases, it may simply involve reducing the dose of the drug in question, or extending the interval between doses to minimize side effects. In other, more serious situations, it may be necessary to suspend the current treatment altogether and look for a therapeutic alternative. For example, if a patient develops acute renal failure following the administration of a nephrotoxic drug, treatment should be stopped immediately, and supportive measures put in place to protect renal function.

Adjustment of care is not limited to changes in drug therapy. It may also include additional interventions to mitigate adverse effects, such as the administration of antihistamines to counter an allergic reaction, gastric protectors to prevent ulcers due to non-steroidal anti-inflammatory drugs, or antiemetic drugs to manage chemotherapy-induced nausea. These complementary interventions are designed to ensure patient comfort and prevent potential complications, while enabling the continuation of the main treatment if it remains necessary and beneficial.

It's also important to communicate these care adjustments to the whole healthcare team to ensure consistent, coordinated management. This includes updating the patient's care plan and holding team meetings, where healthcare professionals discuss the necessary adaptations and how to monitor the effectiveness of the new treatment regimen. This communication ensures that every member of the team is aware of changes and the reasons behind them, enabling increased vigilance and a rapid response in the event of new adverse effects.

Finally, post-adjustment follow-up is crucial to assess the effectiveness of the changes made. Caregivers must continue to monitor the patient closely to ensure that the adverse effect has been resolved and that the new treatment is well tolerated. This monitoring should include regular clinical assessments, laboratory tests if necessary, and ongoing dialogue with the patient to gather feedback and adjust treatment accordingly. If the initial adjustment does not resolve the problem, or if new adverse effects appear, it may be necessary to reassess the situation and call in specialists to explore other therapeutic options.

Chapter 11

Psychogeriatric care in the night shift

- **Understanding the specific needs of elderly patients at night**
  ○ **Sleep disorders in the elderly**

Sleep disorders in the elderly are a common phenomenon that can have a significant impact on their quality of life and overall health. With age, sleep undergoes natural changes, both in terms of quantity and quality. However, these changes can sometimes turn into sleep disorders, exacerbated by various physiological, psychological and environmental factors, making night-time rest less restorative and affecting the vigilance and daytime well-being of the elderly.

One of the most common characteristics of sleep in the elderly is its fragmentation. Sleep often becomes lighter, with less time spent in the deep and REM sleep phases, which are the most restorative. This fragmentation of sleep results in frequent awakenings during the night, often associated with difficulty in getting back to sleep. This phenomenon may be linked to natural changes in the circadian rhythm, which tends to advance with age, but it is also aggravated by medical conditions common to the elderly, such as chronic pain, respiratory disorders such as sleep apnea, or frequent urinary needs due to prostate or kidney problems.

Insomnia, characterized by difficulty falling asleep or staying asleep, is another common sleep disorder among the elderly. Insomnia can be primary, linked to the natural changes of aging, or secondary, resulting from factors such as anxiety, depression, or the use of certain medications that disrupt sleep. Mood disorders, in particular, are often under-diagnosed in the elderly, but can have a profound impact on sleep. Untreated chronic insomnia can lead to daytime fatigue, reduced cognitive ability, and an increased risk of falls and accidents, compromising the quality of life and independence of the elderly.

Restless legs syndrome and periodic limb movements during sleep are also more common with age. These disorders manifest themselves as an unpleasant sensation in the legs and an irresistible urge to move them, which can considerably disrupt sleep. These involuntary movements can lead to repeated awakenings and a feeling of exhaustion on waking. The exact cause of these disorders is not always clear, but they are often associated with iron deficiencies, neurological diseases, or the use of certain medications. Their management requires a thorough medical assessment, and may include nutritional adjustments, modifications to medication regimens, or the use of specific treatments.

Obstructive sleep apnea is another disorder that affects many elderly people. This disorder is characterized by repeated interruptions in breathing during sleep, due to a relaxation of the throat muscles that blocks the airway. These breathing pauses, which can last from a few seconds to a minute, cause micro-awakenings that fragment sleep and lead to excessive daytime sleepiness. Left untreated, sleep apnea increases the risk of cardiovascular disease, hypertension and diabetes, making its diagnosis and management all the more important. Treatment of sleep apnea can include the use of continuous positive airway pressure (CPAP) devices, lifestyle changes such as weight loss and smoking cessation, and in some cases, surgery.

Sleep disorders in the elderly are not just a nocturnal problem; they have a direct impact on the daytime. Lack of restful sleep can lead to persistent fatigue, irritability, reduced attention and concentration, and an increased risk of falls, which can compromise their independence. What's more, poor-quality sleep can exacerbate existing medical conditions, such as heart disease or diabetes, creating a vicious circle where lack of sleep worsens overall health, and vice versa.

Managing sleep disorders in the elderly requires a comprehensive, individualized approach. It begins with a comprehensive assessment of sleep habits, underlying medical conditions, current medications, and psychosocial factors that may be contributing to sleep disorders. Treatment strategies may include behavioral interventions, such as Cognitive Behavioral Therapy for Insomnia

(CBT-I), which has been shown to improve sleep quality. This therapy helps to modify thoughts and behaviors that disrupt sleep, by teaching relaxation techniques, regulating sleep schedules, and improving sleep hygiene.

Improving sleep hygiene is particularly important. It involves creating an environment conducive to sleep and adopting habits that promote quality rest. This includes establishing a regular sleep routine, avoiding caffeine and heavy meals before bedtime, limiting daytime naps, and creating a comfortable, dark, quiet sleep environment. For the elderly, who may spend a lot of time indoors, it's also important to expose themselves to natural light during the day to help regulate their circadian rhythm.

- ○ **The importance of comfort care and night-time reassurance**

The importance of comfort care and night-time reassurance cannot be underestimated in healthcare, particularly for hospitalized patients, the elderly, or those living with chronic illnesses. The night is a particularly vulnerable time for patients, often marked by anxiety, insomnia and feelings of isolation. In this environment, comfort care and reassurance play an essential role in soothing patients, promoting restful sleep, and maintaining a sense of security and well-being.

Night-time comfort care encompasses a wide range of interventions designed to improve patients' physical and emotional well-being at night. This can include simple but essential gestures, such as adjusting bedding to improve comfort, offering an extra pillow, or adjusting the bedroom temperature to make it comfortable. These small attentions can have a significant impact on sleep quality, helping patients to relax and find a comfortable position that reduces pain or discomfort.

Another key aspect of nocturnal comfort care is pain management. Pain can be more intense at night, in the absence of daytime distractions, making sleep difficult for many patients.

Caregivers need to pay particular attention to the assessment and management of nocturnal pain, administering analgesics at the appropriate time or adjusting doses to ensure continuous relief throughout the night. In addition, non-pharmacological techniques such as massage, guided relaxation or the application of hot or cold compresses can be used to ease pain and promote relaxation.

Night-time reassurance, meanwhile, is a fundamental element of emotional support for patients. At night, fears and worries can be heightened, particularly in patients who feel isolated or have concerns about their health or future. Simply being present, listening, and reassuring patients that they are not alone can have a profoundly calming effect. Caregivers need to show empathy and availability, responding to patients' emotional needs in a calm and caring way. A reassuring presence can prevent nocturnal anxiety attacks and help patients feel safe, which is crucial to their overall well-being.

For patients with cognitive disorders, such as dementia, night-time reassurance is particularly important. These patients may feel disoriented or confused at night, which can lead to agitation or disruptive behavior. Reassurance here involves offering temporal and spatial cues, such as reminding them of the time or re-explaining where they are, and using appropriate communication techniques to calm their anxiety. This may include the use of soft light to avoid complete darkness, which can be frightening, or the establishment of a regular night-time routine with which they are familiar.

Comfort care and night-time reassurance also have a direct impact on patients' recovery. Quality sleep is essential for healing, as it allows the body to repair itself, strengthens the immune system, and helps regulate hormones. By providing appropriate comfort care and emotional reassurance, caregivers promote deeper, more restorative sleep, which contributes to better physical and mental recovery for patients. In addition, a soothing nocturnal environment reduces stress, which is known to have negative effects on healing and immune response.

Comfort care and nocturnal reassurance benefit not only patients, but caregivers too. By proactively addressing patients' nocturnal needs, caregivers can prevent many problems that might arise later, such as pain escalations or anxiety attacks, making their work more manageable and less stressful. What's more, knowing they've helped patients have a peaceful and comfortable night boosts caregivers' sense of job satisfaction, which is important for their own well-being and motivation.

Finally, the importance of comfort care and night-time reassurance extends to creating a relationship of trust between patients and caregivers. At night, when patients are most vulnerable, this care creates a bond of trust, showing patients that they are being cared for holistically, with attention and respect. This trust is essential for patients' cooperation in their treatment, for their sense of security, and for their overall experience of care.

- **Managing difficult behavior in psychogeriatrics at night**
  - ○ **Managing confusion and nocturnal agitation**

Managing nocturnal confusion and agitation is a major challenge in patient care, particularly for the elderly, those suffering from cognitive disorders such as dementia, or those hospitalized in unfamiliar surroundings. At night, these patients may experience increased disorientation, agitation and even disruptive behavior, making this a particularly tricky time for caregivers to manage. Understanding the causes of this confusion and implementing appropriate strategies is essential to ensure patients' well-being and maintain a calm, secure environment.

Nocturnal confusion and agitation, often referred to as "sundowning syndrome" or "sundowning", are phenomena in which the cognitive and behavioral symptoms of a person with dementia or neurological disorders intensify at the end of the day or during the night. This can be exacerbated by a number of factors, including fatigue, changes in environmental stimuli, disturbances in the sleep-wake cycle, or darkness itself, which can accentuate feelings of disorientation.

To effectively manage night-time confusion and agitation, it's crucial to create a soothing, structured environment. Lighting plays a key role: soft, indirect light can help reduce fear of the dark and soften shadows that may appear threatening to a confused patient. Avoiding total darkness can reduce disorientation, while respecting the body's need for rest. Caregivers can also use familiar objects, such as photos, blankets or cushions, to create a reassuring setting, reminding the patient of a familiar, safe environment.

A regular night-time routine is also essential to help manage agitation. Maintaining a consistent schedule for evening activities, such as dinner, toileting and bedtime, can provide temporal cues that help stabilize the patient. Routine reassures the patient by providing a predictable structure, reducing the stress and anxiety that can accompany confusion. This routine can be reinforced by soothing activities such as reading a book, listening to soft music, or a relaxation session, all designed to prepare the patient for sleep.

Communication is another vital tool in the management of nocturnal confusion. Caregivers should use simple, clear and reassuring language, avoiding complex terms or multiple instructions that could increase confusion. When a patient is agitated, it's important to speak softly and calmly, using short sentences and repeating information if necessary. Asking open-ended questions and giving the patient time to respond can also help reduce agitation, as it shows that his or her concerns are being heard and taken into account.

Physical contact can be very soothing for some patients. A hand gently placed on the shoulder, gentle pressure on the hand or a hug can convey a sense of security and support, helping to calm the patient. However, it's important to respect individual preferences, as some patients may find physical contact invasive or stressful.

At the same time, it's crucial to assess and treat any underlying medical causes that may be contributing to confusion or nocturnal agitation. For example, a urinary tract infection, untreated pain, hypoglycemia, or medication side effects can all exacerbate confusion. Careful screening and management of these conditions can often significantly reduce nocturnal agitation. In addition, caregivers need to monitor the effect of medications administered at night, particularly sedatives or tranquilizers, which can sometimes have the opposite effect and increase agitation.

It's also important to limit external stimuli that could trigger or aggravate agitation. This includes noise reduction, avoiding loud alarms or background noise which can be disruptive. Similarly, limiting late-night visits and encouraging quiet activities before bedtime can help prepare the patient for a peaceful night. In cases where agitation is severe and persistent, it may be necessary to consult a specialist, such as a neurologist or psychiatrist, to explore specific pharmacological or behavioral interventions.

Finally, the management of confusion and nocturnal agitation must include a supportive approach for the caregivers themselves. Managing these behaviors can be exhausting and emotionally challenging, especially during the nocturnal hours. It is essential that caregivers have access to resources, such as regular breaks, emotional support or stress management counseling, to avoid burnout and ensure that they can continue to provide quality care.

○ **Strategies to minimize the risk of falls and accidents**

Minimizing the risk of falls and accidents, particularly among the elderly and vulnerable, is a key priority in healthcare. Falls are one of the main causes of injury in the elderly, often leading to serious consequences such as fractures, reduced mobility and loss of independence. Implementing effective strategies to prevent these incidents is therefore crucial to preserving patients' safety and quality of life.

The first strategy is to assess each patient's individual risk of falling. This assessment must take into account a range of factors, such as age, general state of health, history of falls, balance disorders, and medications taken by the patient. Certain medications, notably sedatives, antihypertensives or antidepressants, can affect alertness or balance, thus increasing the risk of falling. It is therefore essential that caregivers regularly review prescriptions and consider adjustments in collaboration with the prescribing physician to minimize these risks.

The physical environment in which patients move also plays a major role in preventing falls. It's crucial to ensure that areas where patients move around are safe and free from obstacles. This includes the removal of slippery carpets, trailing cables, and any objects that may impede passage. Floors should be slip-resistant, and areas that are often wet, such as bathrooms, should be equipped with non-slip mats. Lighting is another key factor: sufficient illumination, especially at night, reduces the risk of tripping or disorientation. Nightlights in corridors and bedrooms can help guide patients through the night.

Furniture must also be designed to prevent falls. Beds should be adjusted to the appropriate height to enable the patient to get up and lie down easily, without risk of imbalance. Grab bars or handles should be installed near beds, toilets and showers to provide extra support for movement. Armchairs and chairs should be stable and have sturdy armrests to assist sitting and standing. The use of walkers or canes, adapted to the patient's morphology and needs, can also offer crucial support for people with mobility difficulties.

Another key strategy is to encourage and support regular exercise. Physical activity helps to strengthen muscles, improve balance and coordination, and maintain flexibility, all of which are essential for reducing the risk of falls. Exercise programs designed specifically for the elderly, such as tai chi, walking, or muscle-strengthening exercises, can be particularly beneficial. These exercises should be adapted to each patient's individual abilities and carried out under the supervision of a healthcare professional or physiotherapist, especially in the early stages.

Falls prevention also involves proactive education of patients and their families. Caregivers need to make patients aware of the risks of falls and provide practical advice on how to avoid them. This includes recommendations on wearing appropriate footwear, the importance of getting up slowly after sitting or lying down, and encouragement to ask for help with tasks that could be dangerous. Families also need to be involved in this process, learning how to make the home environment safer and being alert to signs of weakness or imbalance in their loved ones.

Regular monitoring of at-risk patients is also essential. Caregivers must be alert to signs of weakness, dizziness, or other symptoms that could precede a fall. Careful observation, especially of patients who move around at night or have cognitive impairments, can prevent many accidents. In some cases, the use of monitoring devices, such as bed alarms or motion sensors, may be necessary to detect unsafe movement attempts and enable rapid intervention.

Finally, it's important to have a clear plan of action in the event of a fall. Despite all precautions, falls can still occur, and it's crucial that caregivers know how to react to minimize injury and provide appropriate care. This includes first-aid training, immediate assessment of potential injuries, and rapid communication with medical services should the need arise. After a fall, a thorough reassessment of the patient and his or her environment must be carried out to identify causes and adjust prevention strategies.

- **Supporting patients with dementia**
  - **Adapting care to Alzheimer's patients**

Adapting care for patients suffering from Alzheimer's disease is a complex and delicate process, requiring a personalized, empathetic and evolutionary approach. Alzheimer's disease, a common form of dementia, leads to a progressive deterioration in cognitive abilities, affecting memory, thinking, language and daily living skills. For caregivers, whether professionals or family members, adapting care to each stage of the disease is essential to maintain patients' dignity, well-being and quality of life.

One of the most important aspects of adapting care is understanding the unique needs of each patient. Alzheimer's disease progresses differently from person to person, and it is crucial to regularly assess the patient's cognitive and functional abilities. This assessment helps determine the level of assistance needed for activities of daily living, such as dressing, eating, bathing or using the toilet. As the disease progresses, caregivers need to adjust their level of involvement, moving from simple supervision to direct assistance, while respecting the patient's autonomy as far as possible.

Communication is another fundamental pillar of Alzheimer's care. The ability to understand and be understood may diminish over time, but it is essential to maintain a respectful and patient exchange. Caregivers should use simple, clear and concrete language, avoiding complex instructions or open-ended questions that can cause confusion. It's also important to speak slowly, repeating information where necessary, and making sure the patient has understood. Eye contact, a soothing tone of voice, and the use of gestures can also facilitate communication and help establish an emotional connection.

Creating a structured and secure environment is crucial for Alzheimer's patients. People suffering from this disease can feel disorientated, particularly in new or changing environments. Maintaining a stable daily routine helps to reduce anxiety and provide clear temporal cues. Activities should be planned at regular times of the day, and the physical environment should be organized to minimize the risk of confusion or danger. For example, it's helpful to keep personal objects and furniture in the same place, use visual cues such as labels or photos to identify rooms, and limit distractions such as loud noises or bright lights.

Managing disruptive behavior is a common challenge in caring for Alzheimer's patients. Mood swings, agitation, aggression or hallucinations can occur, often triggered by frustration, fear or confusion. It is essential that caregivers approach these behaviors with calm and understanding, seeking to identify the underlying causes rather than repressing the symptoms. For example, an agitated patient may need to go to the bathroom, feel lonely, or be uncomfortable because of the temperature in the room. Offering reassurance, redirecting the patient's attention to a pleasant activity, or modifying the environment to make it more soothing are strategies that can help mitigate these behaviors.

Engaging in meaningful activities is also an essential component of Alzheimer's care. Although cognitive abilities decline, patients can still derive great emotional and mental benefit from participating in activities tailored to their abilities. Creative activities, such as painting or music, gentle physical exercise, such as walking or yoga, and social activities, such as simple games or group discussions, can stimulate the senses, improve mood, and offer a sense of accomplishment. These activities should be chosen according to the patient's interests and abilities, and adjusted over time to remain accessible and enjoyable.

Support for the caregivers themselves is an often overlooked but crucial aspect of caring for patients with Alzheimer's disease. Caring for someone with the disease is physically and emotionally demanding, and it's essential that caregivers have access to supportive resources. This can include specific training on managing the disease, support groups to share experiences and advice, and the possibility of respite to avoid burnout. Adequate support enables caregivers to remain resilient, offer high-quality care and maintain their own well-being.

Finally, end-of-life care for Alzheimer's patients requires a particularly delicate and respectful approach. At this stage, palliative care takes over, with a focus on comfort, pain management and emotional support. Care decisions must be made in collaboration with families, respecting the patient's prior wishes and ensuring that his or her dignity is preserved until the end. The aim is to provide a peaceful, reassuring environment, where the patient can spend his or her final moments surrounded by care and affection.

○ Techniques for maintaining effective communication with disoriented patients

Maintaining effective communication with disoriented patients is an essential skill for caregivers, particularly in the context of caring for the elderly or patients with cognitive disorders such as Alzheimer's disease. Disorientation, whether temporal, spatial or identity-related, can complicate interactions and make patients anxious, frustrated or even agitated. However, with the right techniques, it's possible to strengthen mutual understanding, reduce the patient's stress, and preserve a bond of trust and respect.

One of the first techniques for maintaining effective communication is to create a calm, soothing environment. Disorientation is often exacerbated by distractions, loud noises or chaotic situations. It is therefore crucial to initiate conversation in a setting where the patient can concentrate without distraction. Reducing background noise, such as television or radio, sitting facing the patient to capture his or her attention, and establishing eye contact are important steps in creating a context conducive to exchange. A serene environment helps the patient to feel secure and more willing to communicate.

Using simple, direct language is another key to effective communication with disoriented patients. Short sentences, familiar words and clear instructions help minimize confusion. It's important to avoid idioms, metaphors or abstract concepts that can be misunderstood. For example, rather than saying "I'll check if you need anything," it's clearer to say "I'll see if you're thirsty." Repeating information as necessary, without appearing impatient or frustrated, helps the patient assimilate what is being said. It can also be helpful to ask simple questions that the patient can answer with "yes" or "no", facilitating participation without mentally overloading them.

Patience and active listening are also fundamental to successful communication. Disoriented patients may have difficulty finding the right words, formulating their thoughts, or responding quickly. Caregivers need to be patient, giving patients time to explain what they feel or wish to express, without interrupting or rushing them. Active listening, which involves showing empathy and interest through nods, smiles and encouraging responses, builds the patient's confidence and motivates him or her to continue the conversation. This approach also allows us to pick up on non-verbal signals, such as facial expressions or gestures, which can reveal emotions or needs that words fail to express.

Using visual cues and gestures can greatly facilitate communication with disoriented patients. Simple gestures, such as pointing to a glass of water and asking if the patient is thirsty, or pointing to a chair and inviting the patient to sit down, can help clarify the message. Visual aids, such as photos, pictograms or cards, can also be used to help the patient understand or remember important information. For example, a picture of a clock may remind the patient of mealtime, or a picture of a bed may indicate that it's time to go to bed. These visual cues reduce dependence on words and make communication more accessible for patients with cognitive difficulties.

Adapting tone of voice and body language is also crucial. A soft, calm and reassuring tone of voice is more likely to soothe a disoriented patient than a loud or abrupt one. Facial expressions and posture should reflect a caring, non-threatening attitude, as disoriented patients can be particularly sensitive to non-verbal cues. Leaning slightly towards the patient, smiling, and maintaining benevolent eye contact are gestures that reinforce the feeling of security and trust. It's important to remember that, even if words fail to convey the message, the caregiver's tone and attitude can still communicate support and comfort.

Validation is another effective technique for maintaining positive communication with disoriented patients. Rather than correcting or contradicting a disoriented patient who expresses an erroneous idea or altered perception of reality, it is often more useful to validate his or her feelings. For example, if a patient believes they're in a different place, or talks about a past event as if they were present, instead of telling them they're wrong, the caregiver can say, "This must be an important memory for you." This approach respects the patient's subjective experience, reduces confrontation, and helps maintain an empathetic bond.

Finally, it's essential to adjust expectations and remain flexible when communicating with disoriented patients. Every day can be different, and what works one day may not be as effective the next. Caregivers must be ready to adapt their approach according to the patient's condition, level of fatigue, or mood. The aim is not to force the patient to conform to a communication norm, but to meet the patient where he or she is at, using all available resources to facilitate the exchange.

198

Chapter 12

The Impact of Night Work on Health and Prevention

- **Long-term health effects of night work**
  - **The risk of cardiovascular and metabolic diseases**

Cardiovascular and metabolic diseases represent a major public health issue worldwide, due to their growing prevalence and serious health consequences. These diseases, which include hypertension, coronary heart disease, stroke, type 2 diabetes and obesity, are often interconnected and share common risk factors. Understanding these risks and their impact is essential to preventing these diseases, improving quality of life and reducing associated mortality.

One of the main risk factors for cardiovascular and metabolic diseases is high blood pressure. Hypertension, often referred to as the "silent killer", is a chronic elevation of blood pressure in the arteries, which can damage arterial walls and promote the accumulation of fatty deposits, leading to atherosclerosis. This condition significantly increases the risk of coronary heart disease, stroke and heart failure. Unfortunately, hypertension often presents no noticeable symptoms, which explains why many people are unaware that they suffer from it. Early detection, through regular blood pressure checks, is therefore crucial to managing this risk.

Hypercholesterolemia, or high levels of cholesterol in the blood, is another major risk factor. Cholesterol is a fatty substance essential for the body to function properly, but when present in excess, particularly in the form of low-density lipoproteins (LDL), it can accumulate on artery walls and form atherosclerotic plaques. These plaques reduce the diameter of the arteries, restricting blood flow and increasing the risk of cardiovascular disease, including heart attack and stroke. Regular monitoring of cholesterol levels, combined with a balanced diet and exercise, is essential to control this risk factor.

Type 2 diabetes, a metabolic disease characterized by chronic hyperglycemia due to insulin resistance or insufficient insulin production, is closely linked to cardiovascular disease. Diabetes significantly increases the risk of developing coronary heart disease, stroke or heart failure. Complications of diabetes, such as neuropathy, nephropathy and retinopathy, further exacerbate this risk by affecting the nervous, renal and visual systems. Managing diabetes through strict glycemic control, appropriate diet and regular exercise is therefore essential to prevent associated cardiovascular disease.

Obesity is another major risk factor contributing to the onset of cardiovascular and metabolic diseases. Excess weight, particularly the accumulation of abdominal fat, is associated with increased blood pressure, lipid abnormalities and insulin resistance, creating a breeding ground for the development of diseases such as hypertension, type 2 diabetes and coronary heart disease. Obesity is often the result of several factors, including a sedentary lifestyle, a diet rich in saturated fats and sugars, and genetic factors. Preventing and managing obesity requires a comprehensive approach, including dietary modifications, increased physical activity, and in some cases, medical or surgical intervention.

Lifestyle plays a central role in the prevention of cardiovascular and metabolic diseases. An unbalanced diet, rich in saturated fats, added sugars and salt, contributes to increased weight, blood pressure and cholesterol. Conversely, a diet rich in fruits, vegetables, whole grains and sources of healthy fats, such as omega-3 fatty acids, can reduce these risks. Regular exercise is also crucial to maintaining a healthy weight, improving insulin sensitivity and strengthening the cardiovascular system. Stopping smoking, which damages blood vessels and increases the risk of heart disease, and reducing alcohol consumption, which can contribute to hypertension and obesity, are other important preventive measures.

Chronic stress is an often overlooked but significant factor in the development of cardiovascular and metabolic diseases. Stress can lead to increased blood pressure, unhealthy eating habits, increased physical inactivity, and increased levels of cortisol, a hormone that can promote weight gain and insulin resistance. Stress management through relaxation techniques, meditation, yoga, or recreational activities can help reduce the risk of stress-related cardiovascular and metabolic diseases.

∘ **Chronic sleep disorders and their consequences**
Chronic sleep disorders are a major health problem affecting a growing number of people worldwide. These disorders, which include insomnia, sleep apnea, restless legs syndrome, and circadian rhythm disorder, have profound consequences not only on quality of life, but also on the physical and mental health of individuals. When sleep is disrupted on an ongoing basis, it can lead to a cascade of problems that affect almost every aspect of daily life.

Insomnia, one of the most common chronic sleep disorders, is characterized by difficulty falling asleep, frequent awakenings during the night, or early waking with an inability to fall back asleep. Chronic insomnia can lead to persistent fatigue, irritability and difficulty concentrating. Over time, sleep deprivation can affect cognitive functions, reduce alertness, and impair memory. People suffering from chronic insomnia are also more likely to develop mood disorders, such as anxiety and depression, which can create a vicious circle where stress and anxiety further aggravate sleep problems.

Sleep apnea, another chronic sleep disorder, is characterized by repeated interruptions in breathing during sleep, often accompanied by noisy snoring and feelings of suffocation. These breathing pauses lead to frequent micro-awakenings, preventing deep, restorative sleep. The consequences of sleep apnea are serious, and include a significant increase in the risk of cardiovascular disease, such as hypertension, heart attack and stroke. Untreated sleep apnea is also linked to excessive daytime sleepiness, which increases the risk of road accidents and workplace injuries.

Restless legs syndrome, which causes an irresistible urge to move the legs, especially at night, is another chronic sleep disorder that disrupts nightly rest. Involuntary leg movements can make it difficult to fall asleep and lead to frequent awakenings. This syndrome can lead to chronic fatigue, mood disorders and reduced quality of life, particularly in the elderly, who are more likely to suffer from this disorder.

Circadian rhythm disorders, such as sleep phase delay syndrome, occur when the internal biological clock is out of sync with normal sleep schedules. People with this type of disorder often have trouble falling asleep and waking up at normal times, which disrupts their daily schedule. This can lead to chronic sleep deprivation, affecting performance at work or school, and increasing the risk of mental disorders such as depression and anxiety.

The consequences of chronic sleep disorders extend far beyond fatigue and drowsiness. Sleep deprivation has adverse effects on the immune system, making the body more vulnerable to infection. It also disrupts metabolism, contributing to weight gain and increasing the risk of type 2 diabetes. Chronic sleep deprivation is linked to high levels of inflammation in the body, a major risk factor for many chronic diseases, including cardiovascular disease and certain cancers. In addition, sleep deprivation affects hormonal balance, including the hormones that regulate appetite, which can lead to overeating and obesity.

Sleep also plays an essential role in mental health. Insufficient or poor-quality sleep disrupts emotional regulation, making individuals more susceptible to stress, irritability and depressed mood. The link between sleep and mental health is bidirectional: sleep disorders can aggravate existing mental disorders, and vice versa. For example, people suffering from depression are more likely to experience sleep disorders, and treating insomnia can often improve depressive symptoms.

Managing chronic sleep disorders requires a multidimensional approach. This includes lifestyle changes, such as improving sleep hygiene, regularizing bedtime and wake-up times, and reducing caffeine and alcohol consumption. Behavioral interventions, such as cognitive-behavioral therapy for insomnia (CBT-I), have proved effective in treating many sleep disorders by modifying thoughts and behaviors that disrupt sleep. In some cases, medical treatments, such as continuous positive airway pressure (CPAP) for sleep apnea or medication for restless legs syndrome, may be necessary.

- **Prevention strategies for night nurses**
  - **Balanced diet and sleep management**

A balanced diet and good sleep management are two essential pillars for maintaining optimal health and overall well-being. These two aspects of life are intimately linked, each significantly influencing the other. Understanding and practicing healthy eating habits, while cultivating good sleep practices, can not only improve quality of life, but also prevent many chronic diseases.

Diet plays a key role in sleep quality. What we eat and drink can have a direct impact on our ability to fall asleep, stay asleep, and enjoy restful sleep. For example, foods rich in tryptophan, an amino acid found in foods like turkey, nuts, and milk, are known to promote the production of serotonin, a neurotransmitter that regulates mood and sleep. Serotonin is then converted into melatonin, the sleep hormone, which helps regulate sleep-wake cycles. So eating tryptophan-rich foods, especially at dinnertime, can help prepare the body for a peaceful night's sleep.

On the other hand, certain foods and beverages can impair sleep quality. Caffeine, found in coffee, tea, soft drinks and chocolate, is a stimulant that can interfere with sleep onset and reduce the duration of deep sleep. We recommend avoiding caffeine consumption several hours before bedtime to allow the body to relax naturally. Similarly, while alcohol may initially induce drowsiness, it disrupts the sleep cycle by causing nocturnal awakenings and reducing the time spent in deep sleep. Consuming alcohol before bedtime can therefore lead to poorer quality sleep, even if you fall asleep quickly.

Eating habits, particularly mealtimes, also influence sleep. Eating a heavy meal just before bedtime can cause digestive discomfort, such as heartburn or indigestion, making it difficult to fall asleep. It's best to dine at least two to three hours before bedtime, with a light meal that doesn't overload the digestive system. What's more, a balanced intake of complex carbohydrates, such as those found in whole grains, vegetables and legumes, can stabilize blood sugar levels during the night and avoid awakenings linked to nocturnal hypoglycemia.

The link between diet and sleep goes both ways: just as diet affects sleep, so sleep quality influences food choices. Insufficient or poor-quality sleep can disrupt the hormones that regulate appetite, such as ghrelin and leptin. Lack of sleep increases production of ghrelin, the hormone that stimulates appetite, and decreases production of leptin, the hormone that signals satiety. This hormonal disruption can lead to cravings, particularly for high-calorie, high-sugar foods, and weight gain. Thus, insufficient sleep creates a breeding ground for unhealthy eating behaviors, increasing the risk of obesity and metabolic disorders.

For optimal sleep management, it's important to adopt a regular sleep routine, going to bed and getting up at the same time every day, even at weekends. This regularity reinforces the circadian rhythm, the internal biological clock that regulates the sleep-wake cycle. Good sleep management also includes creating an environment conducive to rest, with a dark, quiet bedroom at a comfortable temperature. Limiting exposure to screens before bedtime is also crucial, as the blue light emitted by electronic devices can inhibit melatonin production and delay sleep onset.

Pre-bedtime relaxation routines, such as reading, meditation or a warm bath, can also prepare the body and mind for sleep. These practices reduce stress and anxiety, two major factors in insomnia, by promoting a state of relaxation that makes it easier to fall asleep. A balanced diet contributes to this relaxation, by providing the nutrients necessary for the production of soothing neurotransmitters, such as magnesium and B vitamins.

◦ The importance of physical activity to offset the effects of night work

The importance of physical activity in offsetting the effects of night work cannot be underestimated, given the many significant health challenges posed by staggered working hours. Night work disrupts the circadian rhythm, the internal biological clock that regulates sleep-wake cycles, which can have a series of negative consequences on physical and mental health. Chronic fatigue, sleep disorders, metabolic imbalances and an increased risk of cardiovascular disease are just some of the potential consequences of night work. In this context, physical activity appears to be a powerful tool for mitigating these effects and promoting overall well-being.

Working at night puts circadian rhythms out of sync, affecting sleep and, in turn, other crucial aspects of health, such as digestion, metabolism and hormone regulation. Regular physical activity can help restore a degree of stability to these disrupted processes. Indeed, exercise helps regulate the sleep-wake cycle by increasing the production of serotonin, a neurotransmitter that plays a key role in regulating mood and sleep. In addition, exercise promotes the production of endorphins, often referred to as "happy hormones", which help reduce stress and anxiety, two aggravating factors for sleep disorders linked to night-time work.

One of the main benefits of physical activity for night workers is its role in managing fatigue and daytime sleepiness. Regular exercise improves sleep quality by increasing the duration of deep sleep phases, which are the most restorative. For night workers, who often have fragmented or poorer-quality sleep, this improvement is particularly valuable. More restorative sleep helps reduce the feeling of fatigue on waking, and improves alertness during working hours. In addition, exercise helps regulate energy metabolism, helping to maintain stable energy levels throughout the day, despite disrupted sleep patterns.

Physical activity also plays a crucial role in the prevention of chronic diseases, an increased risk for night workers. Sleep deprivation and irregular working hours can disrupt fat and sugar metabolism, leading to weight gain, insulin resistance and an increased risk of type 2 diabetes. Regular exercise helps counteract these effects by improving insulin sensitivity, promoting weight loss, and reducing levels of abdominal fat, which is particularly harmful to cardiovascular health. In addition, physical activity is known to lower blood pressure, strengthen the heart and improve blood circulation, thereby reducing the risk of cardiovascular disease, which is more common among night shift workers.

What's more, exercise can play a crucial role in managing stress and preventing burnout, two major concerns for those who work night shifts. Chronic stress, often aggravated by sleep deprivation, can lead to burnout and reduced work performance. Physical activity, in addition to its physical benefits, offers an outlet for mental and emotional stress. Whether through cardio training, yoga, or even outdoor walking, exercise helps to release accumulated tension, improve mood and foster a more positive outlook, even in the face of the challenges of night-time work.

It's important to note that adapting physical activity to night-time schedules is crucial to maximizing its benefits. Night workers need to schedule their exercise sessions at times that don't interfere with their sleep. For example, exercising just before bedtime can disrupt sleep by raising body temperature and stimulating the body. It is therefore advisable to engage in physical activity several hours before bedtime, to allow the body to relax afterwards. Relaxation or stretching exercises, on the other hand, can be performed before bedtime to help calm the body and mind.

Finally, it's essential to stress that physical activity isn't limited to intense workouts. Even everyday movements, such as walking, taking the stairs or doing regular stretches at work, can help offset the effects of night work. These small doses of exercise accumulated throughout the day or night can improve blood circulation, reduce muscle and joint stiffness, and help maintain a more constant energy level.

- **Regular health checks for night nurses**
  - **Specific medical monitoring programs for night workers**

Specific medical monitoring programs for night workers are essential to meet the unique needs of these workers, whose staggered schedules and working conditions can have significant effects on their health. Working at night disrupts circadian rhythms, alters sleep patterns, and can increase the risk of various chronic diseases, such as metabolic disorders, cardiovascular disease, and psychological disorders. This is why it is essential to set up appropriate medical monitoring programs to ensure continuous health surveillance of night workers and prevent complications linked to this type of work.

Above all, these medical monitoring programs must include a thorough initial assessment on taking up the job, to identify the potential risks and specific vulnerabilities of each worker. This assessment includes a full medical examination, including basic tests such as blood pressure measurement, blood analysis to screen for diabetes or high cholesterol, and a cardiovascular examination. An assessment of sleep patterns and mental well-being is also crucial, as night work can profoundly affect these aspects. Identifying early risks enables health recommendations to be adapted, whether through lifestyle adjustments or the implementation of specific preventive measures.

A key aspect of follow-up programs is regular, ongoing monitoring of the health status of night workers. Periodic check-ups, ideally every six months to a year, can detect any deterioration in health that might be linked to night work. These check-ups should include screening tests for cardiovascular disease, sleep assessments to detect possible disorders such as sleep apnea, and examinations to identify early signs of chronic stress or burnout. This continuous monitoring is essential to intervene quickly in the event of emerging health problems, and to adjust working conditions or care recommendations accordingly.

Monitoring mental well-being is another pillar of health programs for night workers. Night work is often associated with increased social isolation, disruption of normal life rhythms and increased stress, all of which can contribute to mental disorders such as anxiety and depression. Medical follow-up programs should therefore include regular consultations with psychologists or mental health counselors, mood and stress assessments, and the establishment of support groups where workers can share their experiences and obtain support. Early detection of mental disorders and provision of adequate support can prevent worsening of symptoms and improve the quality of life of night shift workers.

Monitoring programs should also encourage appropriate sleep management strategies. Night workers should be informed of best practices for optimizing daytime sleep, such as the use of eye masks, blackout curtains, or earplugs to minimize disturbance. Consultations with sleep specialists can be useful for those who have chronic difficulties adapting to night-time schedules. In addition, it is important to educate workers on the importance of maintaining regular sleep schedules, even on days off, to stabilize their biological clock as much as possible.

The integration of programs to promote physical activity is another key element. Regular exercise helps counter many of the negative effects of night work, including improving sleep quality, reducing stress, and preventing cardiovascular and metabolic diseases. Medical follow-up programs can include personalized recommendations for physical activity, adapted to the time constraints of night staff, with exercise suggestions that are easy to integrate into their schedule. Employers can also offer fitness facilities accessible at all times to encourage physical exercise.

Finally, ongoing education on the risks associated with night work and preventive measures is an essential aspect of medical monitoring programs. Night workers need to be well informed about the potential health effects of their schedules and strategies for mitigating them. This can include regular workshops on balanced nutrition, stress management techniques, the importance of hydration, and the effects of caffeine and alcohol on sleep. Ongoing education enables workers to better understand their bodies and take proactive steps to protect their health.

○ **Practical tips for maintaining a healthy lifestyle**
Maintaining a healthy lifestyle is essential for preserving physical and mental health, and for living a fulfilling, energetic life. Adopting healthy habits helps strengthen the immune system, prevent chronic diseases, improve sleep quality, and promote a stable emotional balance. Here are a few practical tips for integrating a balanced lifestyle into your daily routine.

Diet plays a central role in overall health. A balanced diet should be rich in fruits, vegetables, whole grains, lean proteins and healthy fats. Fruits and vegetables provide essential vitamins, minerals and antioxidants that help protect the body against disease. Whole grains, such as brown rice, oats and quinoa, provide long-lasting energy and help regulate blood sugar levels. Lean proteins, found in fish, poultry, legumes, and low-fat dairy products, are crucial for tissue repair and maintaining muscle mass. Healthy fats, such as those found in avocados, nuts and olive oil, are essential for cardiovascular and brain health.

Moderation is also essential when it comes to diet. It's important to limit consumption of added sugar, salt and saturated fats, which can contribute to health problems such as obesity, hypertension and heart disease. Drinking enough water throughout the day is crucial to maintain hydration, support digestion, and promote optimal organ function. It is recommended to drink around eight glasses of water a day, but this requirement may vary according to physical activity and climate.

Physical activity is another pillar of a healthy lifestyle. Regular exercise helps maintain a healthy weight, strengthen muscles and bones, improve mood, and reduce the risk of chronic diseases such as diabetes and heart disease. At least 150 minutes of moderate physical activity per week is recommended, which can include brisk walking, cycling, swimming or fitness classes. Incorporating exercise into your daily routine can be as simple as taking the stairs instead of the elevator, going for a walk after dinner, or indulging in a morning yoga session. The most important thing is to choose activities that you enjoy, making exercise more enjoyable and easier to maintain over the long term.

Sleep is often overlooked, but it's just as crucial to a healthy lifestyle. Quality sleep allows the body to repair itself, regenerate its cells, and consolidate memory and learning. To promote restful sleep, it's essential to maintain a regular bedtime routine, going to bed and getting up at the same time every day, even at weekends. Creating a sleep-friendly environment, with a dark, quiet room at a comfortable temperature, can also help improve the quality of rest. Limiting exposure to screens before bedtime, especially blue light, is crucial to enable the body to produce the sleep hormone melatonin.

Stress management is another key aspect of a healthy lifestyle. Chronic stress can have devastating effects on health, contributing to problems such as hypertension, digestive disorders and depression. So it's important to develop techniques for managing stress effectively. Meditation, deep breathing and the practice of mindfulness are powerful tools for calming the mind and reducing anxiety. Making time for relaxing activities, such as reading, listening to music, or spending time in nature, can also help balance the demands of daily life. In addition, maintaining healthy social relationships and having a strong support network, whether through family, friends or community groups, helps to reduce stress and build emotional resilience.

Work-life balance is also crucial to a healthy lifestyle. It's important to define clear boundaries between work and personal time to avoid overwork and burnout. Taking regular breaks during the working day, disconnecting from professional obligations outside working hours, and making time for pleasurable activities are essential practices for maintaining this balance.

Finally, personal hygiene, including regular hand-washing, proper dental care, and maintaining good body hygiene, is essential to prevent infection and disease. Adherence to these basic hygiene practices is a foundation of daily health, helping to prevent communicable diseases and maintain a clean look and feel.

Chapter 13

The specifics of night work in non-hospital establishments

- **Night work in EHPAD and retirement homes**
  ◦ **The particularities of night care for residents**

Night-time care for residents in healthcare facilities, such as retirement homes, EHPAD, or long-term care units, requires a particular approach, adapted to the specific needs of each individual. Residents are often more vulnerable at night, and the quality of care provided during this period can have a significant impact on their general well-being, health and comfort. Understanding the particularities of night-time care is essential to ensure that residents benefit from continuous, respectful and safe care.

One of the most important aspects of night-time care is managing residents' sleep. Sleep is a fundamental need, especially for the elderly or frail, whose sleep may be naturally disrupted by aging, chronic pain, or specific pathologies. Night carers must be careful to respect residents' sleep cycles, minimizing unnecessary interruptions. This means planning care to minimize nocturnal disturbances, and grouping interventions as far as possible to avoid waking the same resident several times.

However, some interventions are unavoidable, such as changing position to prevent pressure sores, administering necessary medication, or assisting with urgent needs. In these situations, it is essential to act with gentleness and discretion. The use of subdued lighting, soothing voices, and slow, measured gestures helps to reduce the impact of the intervention on the resident's sleep. In addition, caregivers must be trained to assess each resident's condition before intervening, to determine whether the intervention can be delayed or adapted to better respect the resident's sleep.

Managing nocturnal pain is another special feature of night care. At night, pain can become more acute due to the absence of distractions and the slowing down of bodily activities. Residents suffering from chronic pain, such as that associated with osteoarthritis or other conditions, may find their pain intensifies, making sleep difficult. Night caregivers need to be particularly

214

vigilant in this respect, monitoring residents for signs of pain and administering analgesic treatments as prescribed. Active listening is also crucial: residents must feel free to express their discomfort or pain, and know that they can count on a rapid and appropriate response.

Night-time reassurance is an essential component of night-time care, especially for residents suffering from cognitive disorders such as dementia. Night-time can be a source of anxiety, confusion and even agitation for these residents. Feelings of disorientation can be exacerbated by the darkness and silence of the night, making some residents more likely to get up and wander around, increasing the risk of falls. Caregivers need to show patience and empathy, providing appropriate emotional support. This can include simple gestures such as staying by the resident's side for a while, speaking softly to reassure them, or using distraction techniques such as reading a soothing story. Setting up soothing night-time routines, such as playing soft music or using nightlights, can also help reduce night-time anxiety.

Night-time hygiene care, although often perceived as secondary to daytime care, plays a crucial role in residents' comfort. Changing incontinence pads, quick grooming or freshening up are interventions which, if carried out properly, contribute to residents' dignity and well-being. This care must be carried out with particular attention to modesty and communication, explaining each gesture to the resident, even if he or she appears sleepy or disoriented, to maintain a relationship of trust.

Night feeding, although less frequent, may also be necessary for some residents. Caregivers must be ready to respond to specific needs, whether for a light snack recommended by the doctor, or for extra hydration. Warm beverages, such as herbal tea or lukewarm milk, can not only help meet these needs, but also contribute to soothing the resident and easing his or her return to sleep.

Last but not least, constant supervision is one of the major responsibilities of night nurses. It is essential to ensure the safety of residents, especially those at risk of falling, running away or experiencing a sudden deterioration in their state of health. This surveillance must be discreet, so as not to disturb residents unnecessarily, but sufficiently rigorous to enable rapid intervention in case of need. Alarm systems, surveillance monitors and regular rounds are tools which, when used appropriately, combine security with respect for residents' rest.

- **Emergency management in the absence of a permanent medical service**

Managing emergencies in the absence of a permanent medical service represents a major challenge, particularly in healthcare establishments or in isolated settings where healthcare staff are limited or resources are restricted. This situation calls for meticulous preparation, rigorous staff training and effective organization to ensure patient safety and rapid response to critical situations. Although the absence of a permanent medical service may seem worrying, adequate and proactive management can overcome these challenges and ensure that emergencies are treated with the necessary seriousness and efficiency.

The first crucial step in managing emergencies without a permanent medical service is to establish clear, well-defined protocols. These protocols must detail the procedures to be followed in the event of an emergency, precisely indicating the roles and responsibilities of each member of staff present. It is essential that these protocols are regularly reviewed and adapted to the specific needs of the facility or location concerned. They should include guidelines on the initial assessment of the situation, the first steps to be taken, first aid techniques, and the conditions under which it is necessary to contact external emergency services.

Staff training is another key element. In the absence of a permanent medical service, every member of staff must have basic first aid and emergency management skills. This training must be practical, regular and adapted to the different types of emergency situations that may arise. For example, staff must be trained in cardiopulmonary resuscitation (CPR), the use of an automatic external defibrillator (AED), and the management of bleeding, fractures or epileptic seizures. The ability to react quickly and appropriately can mean the difference between life and death in an emergency situation.

In addition to training, regular simulation of emergencies is essential to prepare staff to respond effectively. Simulation exercises not only allow emergency protocols to be put into practice, but also identify any gaps in procedures or staff skills. These simulations should be as realistic as possible, involving a variety of scenarios that may include medical emergencies, fires, or evacuations. Repetition of these exercises builds staff confidence and competence, making reactions smoother and more effective in real-life situations.

Communication is another crucial aspect of emergency management without a permanent medical service. It is essential that staff know how to quickly alert the appropriate authorities and coordinate the response. Emergency numbers, as well as contacts for on-call doctors or emergency medical services, must be easily accessible and well known to all. Communication systems, such as portable radios or cell phones, must be in good working order and accessible at all times. Clear and effective communication means that the necessary resources can be mobilized quickly, and that emergencies can be dealt with in a coordinated manner.

Access to adequate first-aid equipment is also essential. Every facility or site must be equipped with well-stocked first-aid kits that are regularly checked and replenished. These kits should contain everything needed to manage common emergencies, such as bandages, sterile compresses, antiseptics, gloves, scissors and adhesive dressings. In addition, where there is an increased risk of heart attack, a defibrillator should be available, and staff should be trained in its use. Emergency medical equipment must be strategically located, easily accessible and clearly signposted.

In the absence of a permanent medical service, it is also crucial to develop strong relationships with local emergency services, hospitals and clinics. This includes setting up agreements or partnerships that enable rapid access to care when needed. Local emergency services need to be informed about the particularities of the facility or site, the types of emergencies most likely to occur, and the resources available on site. This cooperation ensures better coordination during interventions, facilitating the rapid transfer of patients to appropriate care centers if necessary.

Documentation and evaluation after each emergency incident are also crucial to improving future management. After each emergency, it's important to bring the team together for a debriefing, to discuss what went well and where improvements are needed. This reflection enables protocols to be strengthened, additional training needs to be identified, and resources to be adjusted accordingly. Continuous learning from each incident helps to build team resilience and improve future responses.

Finally, it is essential to maintain constant vigilance and promote a culture of safety within the facility. This means that every member of staff must be alert to signs of deterioration in the health of residents or patients, and must not hesitate to intervene or call for help at the first sign of a possible emergency. Prevention, through careful monitoring and early intervention, can often prevent situations from becoming critical.

- **Night nurses in specialized care centers**
  - **Centers for people with disabilities: specific challenges**

Disability centers are essential places that offer support, care and adapted services to individuals with various types of disability, whether physical, mental, sensory or cognitive. These centers play a crucial role in improving the quality of life of people with disabilities, by providing them with a safe, structured environment conducive to their personal development. However, these facilities face specific challenges that require a particularly attentive, empathetic and innovative approach to meet the complex needs of their residents.

One of the first challenges facing these centers is the diversity of residents' needs. People with disabilities present a wide range of conditions, each requiring personalized and often multidisciplinary care. For example, a person with a motor disability may need assistive devices for mobility, while another with a mental or cognitive disability may require constant support for activities of daily living. This diversity requires centers to have multidisciplinary teams comprising carers, occupational therapists, psychologists, speech therapists and other specialists able to work together to develop individualized care plans. Coordination between these different professionals is crucial to ensure that each resident receives the care and support that meets his or her specific needs.

Another major challenge is infrastructure accessibility. Centers must be designed to be fully accessible for all residents, regardless of their type of disability. This includes not only physical accessibility, with ramps, elevators, wide doors and adapted sanitary facilities, but also sensory and cognitive accessibility. For example, Braille signage for the visually impaired, auditory guidance systems for the hearing impaired, and visual tools or pictograms to help people with cognitive difficulties find their way around are essential. Ensuring all-round accessibility requires ongoing investment in infrastructure, as well as regular training of staff in how to use and maintain these devices effectively.

Communication is also a major challenge in centers for people with disabilities. Many residents may have difficulty expressing their needs, pain or emotions because of their disability. It is therefore essential that staff are trained in alternative communication techniques, such as sign language, the use of communication boards or text-to-speech devices. Establishing effective communication not only helps to better meet the needs of residents, but also enhances their autonomy and active participation in the life of the center. Patience, active listening and empathy are essential qualities for staff, who must constantly adapt the way they interact to each resident's abilities and preferences.

The emotional well-being of residents is another fundamental aspect that requires special attention. People with disabilities can be more vulnerable to isolation, anxiety and depression, especially if they feel misunderstood or marginalized. Centers therefore need to set up programs that promote social inclusion, self-esteem and self-confidence. This can include group activities, creative workshops, art therapy, adapted sports activities, and social outings that enable residents to thrive in a caring and stimulating environment. Psychological support, in the form of regular consultations with psychologists or discussion groups, is also essential to help residents manage their emotions and overcome the challenges associated with their disability.

The involvement of families and loved ones is another specific challenge in the management of centers for people with disabilities. Families play a central role in residents' lives, and their involvement is often a key factor in the success of life projects for people with disabilities. However, families can sometimes feel helpless when faced with the complexity of their loved one's needs, or the administrative and organizational burdens involved. It is therefore crucial that centers establish open and regular communication with families, keeping them informed of their loved one's progress, involving them in important decisions, and offering support in the form of advice, training, or support groups. This collaboration creates a coherent and harmonious environment between the center and the family, reinforcing the well-being and emotional stability of residents.

Managing challenging behavior is another complex aspect of care in centers for people with disabilities. Some residents, because of their disability or associated disorders, may display aggressive, self-aggressive or other forms of disruptive behavior. These situations require a highly specialized approach, based on positive behavioral interventions, a deep understanding of the triggers for these behaviors, and a de-escalation strategy to prevent crises. Staff must be trained to manage these situations calmly, respectfully and effectively, while ensuring the safety of all residents. Collaboration with behavioral specialists and the implementation of personalized management plans are often necessary to reduce these behaviors and improve residents' quality of life.

Finally, the financing and sustainability of centers for people with disabilities are constant challenges. Offering high-quality, adapted and personalized care requires significant resources, both in terms of personnel and infrastructure. Centers often have to navigate between budgetary constraints and the growing demands of regulations and residents' needs. Striking a balance between these factors requires rigorous management, an active search for public and private funding, and ongoing innovation to optimize available resources. This also includes engaging in partnerships with other institutions, NGOs and businesses to develop additional programs and services that enrich the center's offering.

○ Rehabilitation centers: the caregiver's role at night

In rehabilitation centers, the role of the care assistant during the night is essential to ensure continuity of care and patient well-being. Rehabilitation, whether following surgery, treatment for chronic conditions or accidents, is a complex process requiring constant attention, including during the night. The night carer plays a central role in this, providing not only physical care, but also emotional support and attentive monitoring, all of which are essential for patients' progress and safety.

The primary task of the night nurse in a rehabilitation center is to monitor patients. At night, patients are particularly vulnerable, especially those who have difficulty moving around, who are suffering from pain or post-operative complications, or who are disorientated. Caregivers must make regular rounds to ensure that every patient is safe, comfortable and showing no signs of distress. This monitoring is essential to prevent falls, spot early signs of a medical complication, or simply to reassure patients who may feel isolated or anxious in the darkness and silence of the night.

Another crucial aspect of the night carer's role is pain management. Many rehabilitation patients suffer from chronic or acute pain, which can intensify during the night, in the absence of daytime distractions. The caregiver must be alert to signs of pain in patients, even if they do not express it verbally. It is his or her responsibility to administer analgesic treatments as prescribed, monitor their effectiveness, and adjust patient positions to maximize comfort. They must also be able to communicate effectively with patients to understand their level of pain and take the necessary steps to alleviate it, while liaising with the medical team if more extensive intervention is required.

Night-time reassurance is also an essential part of the night carer's job. Night-time can be a time of anxiety for many patients, especially those who are away from home or going through long and arduous periods of rehabilitation. Caregivers need to know how to listen to patients' concerns, answer their questions, and offer them a soothing presence. This reassurance comes in the form of simple gestures, such as adjusting blankets, offering a glass of water, or simply spending a few moments with a worried patient. This emotional support helps to create a secure environment, fostering more peaceful sleep, which is crucial to the healing process.

In addition, the night carer plays a key role in managing hygiene care. Some patients may require dressing changes, skin care to prevent bedsores, or incontinence care. The caregiver must perform these tasks with discretion and gentleness, respecting the patient's dignity while minimizing disruption to sleep. These interventions, although they may seem simple, are fundamental to preventing infection, promoting comfort, and maintaining good hygiene, which is essential for rehabilitation.

The night carer must also be ready to intervene in the event of an emergency. Whether it's a heart attack, fall, respiratory distress or other medical emergency, the caregiver is often the first person to react. They need to be well-trained in first aid, know how to use emergency equipment such as defibrillators, and be able to maintain their composure to manage the situation until on-call medical staff or emergency services arrive. This ability to react quickly and effectively can make the difference in critical situations, ensuring the safety and survival of patients.

Passing on information is another key responsibility of the night carer. At the end of their shift, they must pass on all relevant information to the morning team, including observations on the patient's condition, the care administered, and any special events that occurred during the night. This transmission must be clear and complete to ensure continuity of care and enable the next team to make informed decisions on patient management. Good communication between day and night teams is essential to ensure effective and safe rehabilitation.

Last but not least, the night nurse helps to maintain a calm environment conducive to recovery. At night, rehabilitation centers must remain places of rest and tranquility, where patients can relax and recuperate. The caregiver plays a crucial role in ensuring that noise is kept to a minimum, lights are dimmed, and the general atmosphere is soothing. This setting not only promotes sleep, but also the mental and emotional well-being of patients, which is essential to their recovery.

- **Night missions in psychiatric institutions**
  ◦ **Monitoring and supporting patients in crisis**

Monitoring and supporting patients in crisis are essential and delicate aspects of healthcare, requiring a combination of technical skills, responsiveness and empathy. Seizures can occur unpredictably and take a variety of forms, from psychological crises such as panic attacks or severe anxiety attacks, to medical crises such as epileptic seizures, heart attacks or episodes of extreme agitation in patients with cognitive disorders. Whatever the nature of the crisis, caregivers' priority is to stabilize the situation, protect the patient's safety and provide the necessary support to get them through this critical time.

The first step in managing a seizure is careful monitoring for warning signs. Seizures, although sometimes sudden, are often preceded by symptoms or behaviors that may indicate a deterioration in the patient's condition. For psychological seizures, these signs may include increasing agitation, abrupt mood changes, unusual behavior, or verbal expressions of distress. For medical seizures, the warning signs may be physical, such as tremors, chest pain, breathing difficulties, or changes in consciousness. Constant observation and knowledge of the patient's medical history enable caregivers to intervene early, sometimes even before the crisis becomes critical.

When a crisis occurs, the caregiver's first responsibility is to ensure the safety of the patient and others present. This may involve removing dangerous objects, guiding the patient to a safe position, or calling for back-up if the situation becomes unmanageable on its own. In the case of an epileptic seizure, for example, the patient should be placed on his or her side to avoid airway obstruction, and it is essential not to restrict movement to prevent injury. If the seizure is psychological, such as a severe anxiety attack, it's important to create a calm environment, talk to the patient in a soothing voice, and provide a space where he or she feels safe.

Supporting the patient during a crisis requires clear, simple and reassuring communication. The caregiver must remain calm, regardless of the severity of the situation, as the caregiver's attitude can greatly influence the patient's reaction. Speaking softly, giving simple instructions and offering verbal support can help reduce the patient's anxiety and guide them through the crisis. For example, in the case of a panic attack, the caregiver can encourage the patient to breathe slowly and deeply, focus on a soothing mental image, or engage in simple conversation to divert attention from the fear. The aim is to create a bond of trust, to show the patient that he's not alone and that someone is watching over him.

Managing the physical aspects of the seizure is also essential. If the seizure is linked to a medical condition, such as a heart attack or severe allergic reaction, it's crucial to administer appropriate first aid immediately. This may include the use of emergency medication, such as epinephrine injection in the case of anaphylactic shock, or the implementation of cardiopulmonary resuscitation (CPR) techniques in the case of cardiac arrest. Caregivers must be well-trained in first-aid techniques and the use of emergency equipment, such as automatic external defibrillators (AEDs), and be able to react quickly to stabilize the patient's condition until medical help arrives.

Once the crisis is under control, the patient's support doesn't stop there. The post-crisis phase is often marked by an intense need for reassurance and comfort. The patient may feel vulnerable, confused or exhausted after a crisis, and it's essential that the caregiver remains present to help them regain their composure and understand what has just happened. This can include providing simple explanations of the crisis, listening to the patient's concerns, and following up to prevent future crises. Emotional recovery is just as important as physical recovery, and caring support can make a big difference in how the patient recovers from the episode.

Documenting a crisis is a crucial step in ensuring continuity of care. After each crisis, it is important for the caregiver to accurately record the details of the event, including the symptoms observed, the actions taken, the patient's response, and any medical interventions carried out. This documentation must be shared with the medical team and, if necessary, with the patient's relatives, in order to inform future treatment decisions and adjust care plans to better prevent or manage future crises.

- **Managing safety risks in a psychiatric environment**

Managing safety risks in a psychiatric environment is a complex task requiring constant vigilance, specialized training and a multidimensional approach. Psychiatric environments, whether inpatient units, rehabilitation centers or outpatient facilities, cater for patients with a variety of mental disorders, some of which can lead to unpredictable or dangerous behavior. These behaviours, although often linked to mental suffering, can pose safety risks for the patients themselves, the nursing staff and other residents. Managing these risks effectively is essential to creating a safe, therapeutic environment in which patients can recover and progress.

One of the first steps in managing safety risks is initial and ongoing patient assessment. Every patient admitted to a psychiatric environment must undergo a comprehensive assessment of their mental state, medical history, past behaviors, and any potential risk factors, such as a history of violence, running away, or self-harm. This assessment is used to determine the level of supervision required, and to develop personalized care plans that take into account the specific needs and risks associated with each patient. This assessment is not a one-off process, but needs to be re-evaluated on a regular basis, as the patient's condition and behavior evolve.

Staff training is a key element of safety risk management. Working in a psychiatric environment requires specific skills, including the ability to recognize the warning signs of violent or disruptive behavior, to de-escalate tense situations, and to intervene safely in the event of a crisis. Staff must be trained in non-violent communication techniques, conflict management, and protective physical interventions that minimize the risk of injury to patient and caregiver. Regular training, including simulated emergency situations, is essential to ensure that care teams remain ready to respond appropriately to any unforeseen situation.

The physical layout of the environment also plays a crucial role in risk prevention. Psychiatric units must be designed to minimize potential hazards. This includes eliminating objects or equipment that could be used to injure oneself or others, such as glass mirrors, hooks or cords. Rooms and communal areas should be equipped with secure, non-fixed furniture and discreet monitoring devices that keep an eye on at-risk patients while respecting their privacy. Doors and windows should be secured to prevent escape, but without creating a feeling of confinement, which could aggravate patients' mental state.

Managing aggressive behavior is a specific challenge in psychiatric environments. It is crucial to develop prevention strategies, based on an understanding of individual aggression triggers. For example, some patients may react to specific stimuli, such as noise or lighting, while others may be triggered by interpersonal conflict or frustration. By identifying these triggers, caregivers can adjust the environment and interactions to prevent crises. When aggressive behavior occurs despite these measures, it is essential to intervene quickly to de-escalate the situation, using verbal de-escalation techniques or, if necessary, appropriate physical interventions, while maintaining everyone's safety.

Respect for patients' dignity and rights is a fundamental aspect of risk management in a psychiatric environment. Patients, although they may be in a vulnerable state, have the right to be treated with respect, and their choices must be taken into account as far as possible in care decisions. This means obtaining patients' consent to treatment, informing them in a clear and comprehensible manner, and respecting their confidentiality. At the same time, it is sometimes necessary to take safety measures that may restrict the patient's freedom to protect their life or that of others. In such cases, transparent communication and clear justification of actions taken are essential to maintain a relationship of trust between patient and caregiver.

Interdisciplinary collaboration is also crucial to risk management. Psychiatric environments require close cooperation between various healthcare professionals, including psychiatrists, nurses, psychologists, social workers, and security personnel. This collaboration enables a holistic approach to care, where each team member contributes his or her expertise to develop comprehensive care plans and to intervene effectively in crisis situations. Regular multidisciplinary team meetings, where complex cases are discussed and strategies adjusted, are essential for proactive risk management.

Finally, risk management in the psychiatric environment includes the establishment of clear protocols for emergency situations, such as suicide attempts, assaults or psychotic crises. These protocols must be well known to all staff and regularly updated in line with best practice. After each incident, a debriefing must be organized to analyze what happened, identify what went well and what can be improved, and support staff who may be affected by the event. This feedback process is essential for building team resilience and continuously improving safety procedures.

Conclusion

The Night Nurse's Commitment

- **The irreplaceable role of the night shift orderly**

The role of the nursing auxiliary on night duty is absolutely irreplaceable, so essential is it to the smooth running of care facilities and the well-being of patients. Working at night involves much more than simply looking after sleeping patients. It's a complex mission, imbued with responsibility and dedication, requiring great skill, constant attention, and the ability to handle unforeseen situations in an often silent and dark environment. In reality, the night orderly is the guardian of patients' sleep and well-being, ensuring that their safety, comfort and medical needs are taken care of throughout the night.

The primary mission of the night orderly is to ensure patient safety. During the night, patients are more vulnerable, especially those suffering from chronic illnesses, cognitive disorders or reduced mobility. The caregiver must monitor vital signs, be alert to changes in health status, and intervene rapidly in the event of deterioration. For example, it may be necessary to monitor the breathing of a patient with a respiratory ailment, check the temperature of a febrile patient, or react to an alarm signaling a drop in blood pressure. This constant, discreet but vigilant monitoring ensures that patients are protected from nocturnal risks, and that any emergencies are dealt with immediately.

Patient comfort is another key dimension of the night carer's work. Sleep is a crucial time for physical and mental recovery, and the caregiver plays an important role in creating an environment conducive to rest. This can include simple but essential tasks, such as adjusting patients' position to prevent bedsores, making sure they are well covered, or bringing them a glass of water if they wake up. For patients suffering from chronic pain, the night carer needs to be particularly vigilant and responsive, administering prescribed analgesics or finding non-pharmacological means of relieving discomfort, such as gentle massage or the application of warm compresses.

The role of the night carer is not limited to physical care. It also includes an emotional and psychological dimension. At night, some patients may feel lonely, anxious or disoriented, especially in a hospital or nursing home environment, far from their familiar surroundings. The caregiver must be able to recognize these signs of distress and offer appropriate support. This can take the form of a reassuring presence, a soothing word, or simply holding a patient's hand to calm them down. These gestures, though simple, have a profound impact on patients' well-being, offering them a sense of security and comfort at a time when they feel particularly vulnerable.

Night nurses also need to be highly autonomous and able to make quick decisions. Unlike daytime services, where medical teams are often larger and doctors more readily available, at night resources are more limited. The caregiver often has to manage urgent situations independently, while knowing when it's necessary to contact a nurse or doctor on call. For example, if a patient falls, the caregiver must quickly assess the seriousness of the situation, administer first aid, and decide whether medical intervention is required. This ability to act quickly and effectively is essential for patient safety and continuity of care throughout the night.

Continuity of care is another fundamental aspect of the nursing auxiliary's role on night duty. Although the night is a time of rest, care must continue without interruption. This includes monitoring infusions, administering nocturnal medication, managing medical devices such as urinary catheters, and responding to patients' immediate needs. The caregiver must also ensure that relevant information is passed on to the day team when changing shifts. This is crucial to ensure that care is coordinated, and that the day teams are fully informed of patient status and interventions carried out during the night.

Finally, night work requires the caregiver to have a particular ability to manage circadian rhythms and maintain their own well-being. Working at night can disrupt the natural sleep cycle and affect physical and mental health. Caregivers must therefore be able to manage their rest time, maintain a balanced diet, and find ways to relax and recharge during the day. This self-management is essential if they are to remain alert and efficient during night-time working hours, when fatigue can be a dangerous enemy.

- **A call to vocation: the importance of empathy and dedication**

A call to vocation, particularly in the care and support professions, is an invitation to embrace deeply human values such as empathy and dedication. These qualities, far more than mere technical skills, are at the heart of what distinguishes a committed healthcare professional or carer, capable of transforming care into a true mission of life. Empathy and dedication are not just desirable qualities, but essential elements that nurture and sustain a vocation in demanding professions where the well-being of others is central.

Empathy is the ability to understand and share another person's feelings. In the context of care, it manifests itself in attentive listening, a sincere understanding of patients' pains, fears and needs, and an appropriate, benevolent response. Empathy goes beyond simple sympathy; it involves putting oneself in the other person's shoes, feeling what they're feeling, and using this understanding to offer support that goes beyond the strictly medical. An empathetic caregiver is not just a care technician, but a companion to vulnerable people, offering not just physical care, but a comforting and reassuring presence.

Dedication, on the other hand, is a deep and abiding commitment to serving others, often to the detriment of one's own interests or comfort. In the care professions, dedication translates into constant availability, a willingness to go beyond expectations to meet patients' needs, and an ability to persevere even in the face of difficult or exhausting situations. A dedicated caregiver is one who stays at the bedside of a restless patient, even after a long

232

day, who takes the time to ensure that every detail is taken care of, and who finds the strength to smile and comfort, even when he or she is tired. This dedication is not just a professional requirement, but a manifestation of vocation, where the well-being of others becomes a priority that guides every action.

The importance of empathy and dedication in the care professions cannot be overstated. These qualities are what humanize care, what transform a clinical interaction into a relationship of trust and mutual respect. Patients, whether in hospitals, nursing homes or at home, are not just looking for medical care; they're looking for understanding, compassion, and reassurance that those around them genuinely care about their well-being. Empathy enables us to make this connection, to look beyond symptoms and diagnoses to understand the whole person, with his or her emotions, fears and hopes.

Dedication, on the other hand, is the force that sustains empathy, that drives the caregiver to keep offering that support, day after day, even when the challenges are many and the rewards sometimes invisible. Dedication is the commitment to always do one's best, to learn, to improve, and to never give up, even when the task seems overwhelming. It's this inner strength that enables caregivers to overcome moments of doubt, fatigue or discouragement, and continue to offer care of impeccable quality.

But empathy and dedication are not qualities that can be cultivated on their own; they are nurtured by vocation, by that inner call that drives a person to choose a caring profession, not out of mere obligation or for material reasons, but out of a deep desire to make a difference in the lives of others. This vocation is what transforms challenges into learning opportunities, hardships into moments of growth, and daily work into a life mission. It gives meaning to effort, purpose to action, and deep satisfaction in seeing the positive impact of one's work on the lives of others.

By cultivating empathy and dedication, caregivers don't just demonstrate competence; they embody the highest values of humanity, those of altruism, compassion and solidarity. They show that caring for others is much more than a job; it's a moral commitment, an act of love, and an expression of the best of who we are as human beings.

- **Future prospects for night nurses**

The future prospects for future night nurses are rich in promise, but also marked by challenges that demand continuous adaptation and a willingness to innovate. As the need for healthcare continues to grow, not least due to the aging of the population and the increase in chronic illnesses, the role of night nurses is becoming increasingly crucial. These professionals play an indispensable role in the continuity of care, providing a reassuring presence and essential care during the quietest but often most vulnerable hours for patients. The future of this profession lies in the growing recognition of its importance, the evolution of care practices, and the integration of new technologies.

One of the first prospects for future night nurses is increased recognition of their role in the healthcare system. Traditionally, night work has been perceived as less visible and sometimes less valued than day work. However, this perception is changing as the importance of continuous care and the quality of care provided during the night becomes better understood. Night nurses not only ensure patient safety and comfort, they also play a crucial role in monitoring vital signs, managing pain, and responding to emergencies. Increased recognition could mean better training, wider career opportunities, and fairer pay for these professionals.

The evolution of care practices is another important perspective for future night care assistants. As models of care become increasingly patient-centered, night orderlies will be called upon to play a more active role in the planning and implementation of individualized care. This involves greater collaboration with interdisciplinary teams, increased participation in clinical decision-making, and expanded responsibility for managing complex care. For example, night nurses could be increasingly involved in the management of palliative care, where an empathetic and personalized approach is essential to accompany end-of-life patients and their families.

Technology will also play a key role in the future of night care assistants. Technological advances, such as remote monitoring devices, digital communication tools, and electronic care management systems, will transform the way night care is delivered. Night caregivers will need to familiarize themselves with these technologies, which can facilitate patient monitoring, improve communication between care teams, and offer real-time data for more informed decision-making. For example, smart sensors can monitor a patient's vitals and instantly alert staff to critical changes, enabling rapid intervention. These technologies, while not replacing the human dimension of care, will enhance the efficiency and safety of night-time care.

In addition, ongoing training will be a key issue for future night care assistants. As the demands of the profession evolve, it will be crucial for these professionals to keep up to date with the latest care practices, technological innovations, and patient-centered approaches. Training programs will need to incorporate specific modules on night care, emergency management, and the use of new technologies. In addition, training in stress management and resilience will be essential to help night carers cope with the specific challenges of their work, such as staggered hours and exposure to crisis situations.

However, the human dimension of the work carried out by night nurses will remain at the heart of their profession, whatever the technological and practical developments. Accompanying patients through the night requires a particular sensitivity, an ability to reassure and soothe, and constant attention to patients' often unspoken needs. In the future, night nurses must continue to cultivate these qualities, while adapting to the new realities of the profession. They will also need to be advocates of patient well-being, ensuring that their physical, emotional and psychological needs are addressed holistically.

Finally, the future of night nurses will also be marked by greater attention to their own well-being. Working at night presents specific challenges, particularly in terms of physical and mental health, linked to circadian rhythm disruption, fatigue, and isolation. Healthcare facilities will need to put in place strategies to support night carers, such as occupational health programs, break arrangements, and psychological support initiatives. Recognition of the importance of their work should also be reflected in working conditions that promote their well-being and resilience, so that they can continue to provide quality care.

Appendices : Practical tools and resources

- **Practical sheets for the night shift**
  - **Sample written transmissions for service handover**

Written shift handover templates are essential tools for ensuring continuity of care in healthcare facilities. These transmissions, carried out at each shift change, enable crucial information on patient condition, interventions performed, and important observations to be passed on to the next team. Efficient, clear and structured transmission is fundamental to avoiding errors, ensuring consistent follow-up care, and maintaining a high level of quality in patient care.

The first key element of a written transmission model is clarity of information. Each transmission should begin with the patient's identification data: surname, first name, age, and room or bed number. This ensures that information is correctly assigned and avoids confusion between patients. Next, it's important to summarize the patient's general condition, mentioning their main diagnosis, comorbidities, and any recent major interventions, such as operations or changes in treatment. This overview helps the next team to quickly understand the patient's clinical context.

A section dedicated to observations during the night or day is crucial. This involves noting any relevant observations made during the shift, whether these be changes in vital signs, the appearance of new symptoms, or unusual behaviors. For example, if a patient showed signs of agitation, had difficulty breathing, or expressed particular pain, these details should be clearly documented. The importance of these observations lies in their ability to alert the next team to potentially critical developments in the patient's condition, enabling a rapid and appropriate response.

The written report must also include an update on the care provided during the shift. This includes basic care, such as medication administration, hygiene care or dressing changes, as well as more specific care, such as interventions linked to medical devices (catheters, infusions) or technical acts (sampling, injections). Each treatment should be described concisely but precisely, noting times of administration, dosages, and any reactions observed in the patient. This section ensures that all necessary care has been taken, and that no important details have been omitted.

Specific instructions to be passed on to the next team are another important aspect of written transmissions. These may be specific instructions for monitoring a patient, such as close monitoring of vital signs, attention to a wound, or the need to carry out a complementary examination. These instructions must be written explicitly and unambiguously, so that the next team knows exactly what is expected of them. For example, it might say: "Monitor patient's heart rate closely in room 202, risk of tachycardia observed last night."

Another crucial element to include is the status of current treatments. This means specifying the treatments administered, their efficacy, and any recent modifications. If a drug has been modified, stopped or added, this information must be clearly stated, along with the reasons for the change. In addition, reactions to treatments, whether positive or negative, must be noted so that the next team can adjust care accordingly. For example: "Patient tolerated adjustment of antihypertensive treatment well, blood pressure stable overnight."

Written transmissions should also mention any interactions with family or close friends. This includes any information conveyed to families, the questions or concerns they raised, and the answers given. This is particularly important in situations where families play an active role in the patient's care, or where a shared decision is required. Documenting these exchanges ensures that the next team is aware of everything that has been discussed and of the families' expectations.

Last but not least, it is essential that all written transmissions are signed and dated by the healthcare professional drafting them. This signature attests to the accuracy and completeness of the information transmitted, and lets you know who to contact if clarification is needed. The date and time of transmission are also important to contextualize the information and ensure that care is properly monitored over time.

◦ **Night surveillance grids**

Night-time monitoring grids are essential tools in healthcare establishments to ensure continuous, organized and systematic monitoring of patients during the night. They enable caregivers to rigorously monitor patients' state of health, rapidly detect any abnormalities, and document the care and interventions carried out. They play a crucial role in preventing complications and ensuring patient safety during hours when vigilance is particularly necessary.

A well-designed nighttime monitoring grid starts with basic patient information, such as surname, first name, age, room number and main diagnosis. This information is essential to quickly identify each patient and to contextualize observations made during the night. At the start of the night, a brief summary of the patient's condition and specific points of attention (such as close monitoring of a wound or a tendency to disorientation) can be noted, providing a clear framework for future monitoring.

The nocturnal monitoring grid is then organized into different sections covering the key aspects of monitoring. One of the main sections is dedicated to vital signs, including temperature, blood pressure, heart rate and oxygen saturation. These parameters are measured at regular intervals, according to the patient's specific needs, and accurately recorded. An abnormal evolution of these vital signs can indicate a deterioration in the patient's state of health, and the grid enables these variations to be tracked over several hours, facilitating rapid intervention if necessary.

Another important section concerns the patient's state of consciousness and behavior. For patients in intensive care, post-operatively, or with cognitive disorders, it is crucial to monitor any changes in state of consciousness, whether confusion, excessive drowsiness or agitation. These observations should be documented in the chart with clear, precise descriptions, enabling any significant changes to be identified quickly, which may require medical assessment or adaptation of care.

Pain management is another aspect covered by night-time monitoring grids. Pain, which is often exacerbated at night, must be assessed regularly, using appropriate pain scales, and any intervention, whether or not it involves medication, must be recorded. For example, if an analgesic is administered, it is important to document the time, dose and effect observed, to ensure adequate follow-up and to inform the daytime team of the evolution of the situation.

Nursing and hygiene care are also included in the monitoring grids. Caregivers must note interventions such as position changes to prevent pressure sores, incontinence care, or any assistance provided for the patient's comfort, such as adjusting sheets or pillows. These notes ensure that all necessary care has been taken, and that the patient has received continuous attention throughout the night.

For patients undergoing specific treatments, such as infusions, catheters or drains, a section of the grid is dedicated to monitoring these devices. It is essential to regularly check that they are working properly, to note any anomalies (such as leakage or displacement), and to ensure that the volumes administered correspond to the prescriptions. All interventions and adjustments must be recorded, enabling full traceability of the care provided.

Finally, the night-time monitoring grid should include a space for free comments, where caregivers can note any particular observations that don't fit into the predefined sections, but could be important for continuity of care. This could include interactions with the patient, reactions to certain care, or comments on the patient's environment, such as noise or light levels.

The night-time monitoring charts are then passed on to the next team when the shift is handed over. They are an invaluable reference document, enabling clear and effective communication on the condition of patients, the interventions carried out, and the points of vigilance to be pursued. This written transmission, combined with oral transmissions, ensures that the day team has all the information it needs to continue offering quality care.

- **Useful addresses and online resources for caregivers**

For new and experienced caregivers alike, having access to useful addresses and online resources is essential for training, keeping up to date with the latest practices, and finding support in their day-to-day practice. These resources offer access to a wealth of information, tools and practical advice, reinforcing the skills and confidence of professionals in a field where knowledge and techniques are constantly evolving.

1. Training organizations and professional associations

Training organizations specializing in the healthcare field are essential partners for nursing assistants. Among them, the Association Nationale des Aides-Soignants (ANAS) offers ongoing training courses, workshops and conferences to help caregivers improve their skills and keep up to date with new techniques and regulations. Aides-soignants can also join this association to benefit from a professional network and career support.

Another key organization is the Agence nationale du développement professionnel continu (ANDPC), which offers online and face-to-face training programs. These programs are often financed for healthcare professionals, enabling caregivers to train at no personal cost. Continuous training is essential to remain competent in a constantly evolving profession.

2. Online resources for training and information

Caregivers can also benefit from numerous online resources offering educational content and up-to-date information. The *Infirmiers.com* website, although primarily aimed at nurses, features a section dedicated to caregivers with articles, practical fact sheets, and discussion forums where professionals can share their experiences and ask questions.

Another useful site is *Santé sur le Net*, which offers reliable medical information and thematic dossiers on various pathologies and care techniques. This site is particularly useful for caregivers who wish to deepen their medical knowledge or better understand the health conditions of the patients they care for.

3. Tools and applications for daily practice

Caregivers can also take advantage of digital tools to facilitate their day-to-day work. For example, the *MediSafe* mobile app enables them to manage medication, track patient treatment and receive reminders to take their medication. This app is particularly useful for caregivers who manage complex treatments and want to make sure they don't forget anything.

The *Rescue* app is another valuable tool, offering first aid training directly on the smartphone. The app enables caregivers to regularly review first aid techniques and prepare for rapid intervention in the event of an emergency.

4. Online communities and professional social networks

Online communities and professional social networks are excellent ways for caregivers to connect with their peers, share experiences and find support. On Facebook, there are several groups dedicated to caregivers, such as "Aides-Soignants de France", where members exchange advice, job offers and feedback on different aspects of their profession.

LinkedIn is another important network for caregivers wishing to develop their professional network. By following healthcare organization pages or joining professional discussion groups, caregivers can keep abreast of developments in the sector, training opportunities, and best practices.

5. Online guides and manuals

To deepen their knowledge, caregivers can access online guides and manuals. The *Doctissimo* website offers comprehensive guides on caring for the elderly, basic care techniques, and good hygiene and safety practices. These guides are often written by healthcare professionals and are regularly updated to reflect the latest recommendations.

Another useful guide is the *Guide de l'Aide-Soignant*, available in digital format on platforms such as Amazon or Fnac. This reference book covers all aspects of the profession, from the basics of care to managing complex situations. It is ideal for nursing assistants in training or for those wishing to consolidate their knowledge.

6. Wellness and stress management resources

The work of a caregiver is demanding and can sometimes be a source of stress and burnout. To help caregivers manage their well-being, sites like *Psycom* offer resources on stress management, relaxation techniques, and advice on preventing burn-out. This site also offers information on psychological support services, which can be useful for caregivers in difficulty.

The *Headspace* website offers meditation and mindfulness programs specially designed for healthcare professionals. These programs can help caregivers stay calm and focused, even in stressful work environments.

- **Bibliographical references and specialized articles**

Bibliographical references and specialized articles play a crucial role in the training and professional development of nursing assistants. These resources help to deepen knowledge, keep abreast of the latest advances in the healthcare field, and reinforce the skills needed to provide quality care. For caregivers, access to a well-chosen bibliography and specialized articles is essential for understanding care practices, evolving medical protocols and the ethical issues involved in their profession.

1. Reference books for nurses' aides

Reference books are indispensable tools for nursing assistants, providing comprehensive information on both the theoretical and practical aspects of their profession. Among the must-have books is the *Guide de l'Aide-Soignant*, often considered a bible for professionals in training. It covers a wide range of topics, from basic care techniques to more complex protocols, patient communication and emergency management. The guide is designed to be used both as a training aid and as a reference in daily practice.

Another key book is *Techniques de soins aux personnes âgées et dépendantes* by Monique Villeneuve, which focuses specifically on geriatric care. This book explores in depth the particular needs of the elderly, offering practical advice and techniques adapted to their care. It also addresses the psychological and social aspects of caring for the elderly, making it an invaluable resource for caregivers working in nursing homes or geriatric wards.

2. Trade magazines and periodicals

Specialized journals are another essential source of information for caregivers. Publications such as *La Revue de l'Infirmière* et *Soins Aides-Soignantes* feature articles written by healthcare professionals, researchers and experts in the field. These journals cover a wide range of topics, from new care methods to case studies and legislative and regulatory developments. This enables caregivers to keep up to date with the latest practices and innovations, while enriching their understanding of the challenges they face in their day-to-day work.

In addition, some magazines such as *Soins* offer themed issues that delve deeper into specific topics, such as palliative care, pain management, or chronic disease management. These specialized articles enable caregivers to develop expertise in particular areas, helping them to respond more effectively to patients' specific needs.

3. Scientific articles and clinical research

Scientific articles and clinical research are also valuable resources for nursing assistants wishing to deepen their knowledge and understand the scientific underpinnings of care practices. Online databases such as *PubMed* and *Cairn.info* offer access to thousands of scientific articles, covering all aspects of health and nursing. Caregivers can use these resources to search for specific information, such as the latest studies on pain management, the effects of treatments, or best practices in infection prevention.

Reading scientific articles also enables caregivers to develop critical thinking skills, evaluating the evidence behind care practices and staying abreast of current debates in the healthcare field. For example, a recent article published in *The Lancet* on the impact of patient-centered care in intensive care units could offer valuable insights into how to improve the quality of care in the most complex settings.

4. Specialized books on ethics and communication

Ethics is a fundamental aspect of the caregiver's profession, and specialist books such as *Ethique et déontologie pour les aides-soignants* by Geneviève Gay provide a framework for understanding the ethical dilemmas faced by caregivers. This book tackles delicate issues such as respect for patient dignity, informed consent and confidentiality, providing tools for navigating these situations with integrity and compassion.

Communication is also a key issue for caregivers, and books such as Philippe Jeammet's *Communiquer avec le patient* provide strategies for improving interactions with patients, especially those who are vulnerable or in dependent situations. Good communication is essential for establishing a relationship of trust with patients, understanding their needs, and offering them quality care.

5. Access to online resources and digital libraries

Finally, caregivers can access numerous online resources and digital libraries to enrich their knowledge. Platforms such as *Google Scholar* enable users to search for academic articles and theses on specific subjects, while sites such as *OpenEdition* offer free access to scientific publications in the humanities and social sciences, including healthcare.

The digital libraries of major healthcare institutions, such as the Institut National de la Santé et de la Recherche Médicale (INSERM), are also valuable resources. These platforms offer access to a vast collection of books, articles and research reports, often freely available, enabling caregivers to keep up to date with the latest knowledge.

www.ingramcontent.com/pod-product-compliance
Lightning Source LLC
Chambersburg PA
CBHW072143290526
45794CB00004B/1406